An Introduction to Stata for Health Researchers

Researchers

Second Edition

An Introduction to Stata for Health Researchers

Second Edition

SVEND JUUL
Institute of Public Health
Department of Epidemiology
Aarhus University
Aarhus, Denmark

A Stata Press Publication
StataCorp LP
College Station, Texas

Published by Stata Press, 4905 Lakeway Drive, College Station, Texas 77845
Typeset in LaTeX 2_ε
Printed in the United States of America

10 9 8 7 6 5 4 3 2 1

ISBN-10: 1-59718-044-0
ISBN-13: 978-1-59718-044-3

Contents

Tables

Figures

Preface to the second edition

This second edition updates the first edition (written to support Stata 9) to reflect the changes in Stata 10, which was released in June 2007. Important new elements are the new date and time variables, the Graph Editor, exact logistic and Poisson regression, and power analysis for survival data.

The main structure of this edition is the same as the first edition except for one element: the first edition included a few exercises, while this second edition includes many. The exercises are intended to assist your learning the basics of Stata. You will find the exercises in chapter 20. Suggested solutions to the exercises are not included in the book, but are available at the book's web site, http://www.stata-press.com/books/ishr2.html.

The expansion of the section with exercises was suggested by several users of the first edition, and a few other changes were also inspired by suggestions from users. User reactions are very welcome and can be a good inspiration to further improvements, so please feel free to send comments to sj@soci.au.dk.

Bill Rising at StataCorp gave several useful suggestions and has been very helpful in the production of this book.

Aarhus, Denmark   Svend Juul
June 2008

Preface to the first edition

The main intent of this book is *empowerment*: I want to help you benefit from using Stata in your own research. Your research is probably demanding enough as it is, but to many researchers, the technicalities of data management and analysis can cause major problems — sometimes overwhelming problems. Stata has the tools you need. The purpose of this book is to help you use them.

Stata is a versatile program aimed at data management, statistical analysis, and graphics for research. It is dynamic, too, with new and improved tools being added by Stata monthly, and with contributions from an enthusiastic user community daily. This rapid development pace may make the inexperienced user feel a bit lost in what may initially look like a huge jungle. I want to help you become familiar with the basics and benefit from some of the more advanced analytic tools. I will not be able to demonstrate everything Stata can do, but I hope to help you get started — and more.

This book is an introduction, written for the newcomer who has little or no experience with Stata. But it will also be a valuable companion for more-advanced users. Although I wrote the book to meet the newcomer's needs, I chose to build it systematically, e.g., by putting everything about calculations in one chapter, from the basics to the more complex stuff. This systematic structure makes it easy to locate the information you need. Some of the exercises are aimed at beginners.

The systematic approach also means that you should not try to understand or learn everything in the sequence in which it is presented, e.g., in chapter 4 on command syntax. But now that you know it is there, when you have a general question on Stata's grammar, you can look in that chapter to find the answer.

The book's primary audience is people working with health research. When selecting which data management and analysis tools to demonstrate, I chose the tools that, in my experience, are most often used in health research. But there is much more to it than what is shown in this book. Stata has hundreds of commands. I discuss a few of them and point to some other commands that might be useful to you. In addition to the official Stata commands, there are a thousand user-generated contributions. I point to a few of them, too, and demonstrate how to find and use them.

Writing this book has been a joy (mostly). One of the best parts of the experience has been the enthusiastic discussions I have had with people at StataCorp. In particular, Alan Riley, Vince Wiggins, and Bennet Fauber have given a lot of useful input, and Terri Schroeder and Lisa Gilmore have skillfully prepared the manuscript for printing. The most important input, however, was from the students I taught and supervised.

If you believe you have discovered an error, or if you have a suggestion for improving the book, please send an email to sj@soci.au.dk.

Aarhus, Denmark   Svend Juul
February 2006

Online supplements

This book has several online resources associated with it, which you can find at

http://www.stata-press.com/books/ishr2.html

Resources on this web site include

- datasets.
- programs, such as those for easy handling of output (see section 17.3).
- a do-file for each graph shown. I sometimes show only the minimal command needed to display a graph. The corresponding do-file includes all the options used to obtain the final graph.
- a link to supplementary materials.
- errors and corrections. These (if any) will be shown in an *Errata* section. If you believe you have discovered an error, or if you have a suggestion for improving the book, please send an email to sj@soci.au.dk. Do not use this address to obtain help; for help, see chapter 2.

There may be other resources placed on the web site after this book goes to press, so visit it to see what else appears there.

Notations in this book

Stata commands and the corresponding output are generally shown in these typefaces:

```
. webuse lowbirth.dta
(Applied Logistic Regression, Hosmer & Lemeshow)
. keep pairid low smoke
. list in 1/4, sepby(pairid)
```

	pairid	low	smoke
1.	1	0	0
2.	1	1	1
3.	2	0	0
4.	2	1	0

The commands you can enter are shown in boldface and are preceded by a period that represents Stata's command prompt. Do not type the period.

When referring to menu items, I use a sans serif font, for example

Statistics ▷ Summaries, tables, and tests ▷ Nonparametric tests of hypotheses

I use slant font to show keystrokes, such as *Ctrl+C* and *Enter*.

1 Getting started

This chapter describes how to install, update, and customize Stata and demonstrates the use of various windows.

Before starting to work with Stata, you must know your operating system and make some decisions about how to use it. Actually, this requirement applies to any software, but it is especially critical when you work with your own data, which may have been collected at great expense. I describe primarily how to work in Windows, and I refer to the *Getting Started with Stata for Windows* manual ([GSW]). However, the other *Getting Started* ([GS]) manuals are organized similarly, and users of other platforms can use the relevant [GS] manual.

First, you must decide where to put your files, such as datasets and other documents. The newer Windows versions initially suggest that you store files somewhere along a long branch starting with Documents and Settings. I recommend that you choose a simpler structure and store your documents in subfolders under your personal main folder. In this book, we will store files in subfolders of C:\docs. For more specific advice on how to work with Windows, see chapter 21.

In the book's examples, I assume that you downloaded the datasets associated with the book to C:\docs\ishr2, but you can store them where you wish; for instructions, see http://www.stata-press.com/data/ishr2.html.

> In section 20.1, you find exercises related to this chapter. If you are a newcomer to Stata, these exercises will help you get started.

1.1 Installing and updating Stata

Installing

Insert the installation CD and follow the instructions. [GSW] **1 Installation** gives more details, if needed.

Stata suggests that you use C:\data as the default working directory. I recommend that you choose C:\docs or whatever your personal main folder is; see section 1.3.

Before we get started, you should update Stata.

Updating

It is important that you update Stata before you proceed. StataCorp regularly releases free enhancements and bug fixes to Stata. It is a good idea to make sure that you have the very latest set of changes. To obtain these, you must be connected to the Internet. For more about updating, see [GSW] **20 Updating and extending Stata — Internet functionality** and [R] **update**.

From Stata's menu bar, select

Help ▷ Official Updates

A Viewer window opens, showing you the dates for the executable (the main program, here wsestata.exe[1]) and ado-files currently installed. See figure 1.1.

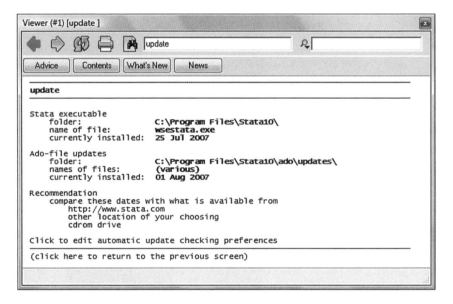

Figure 1.1. Viewer window showing dates of currently installed files

> **Windows Vista users:** The default Vista permission settings do not allow applications write permissions to their respective install directories, even if you are logged in to a machine as administrator. Stata needs these permissions to update. To get around the problem, you must right-click on the Stata executable in the Stata install directory and select **Run as Administrator**. Then you can update as described in this section.

---

1. wsestata.exe is the name of the executable for Stata/SE. For Stata/IC, it is wstata.exe, and for Small Stata, it is wsmstata.exe. If you use a Macintosh or Unix computer, the names will differ slightly.

Follow the recommendation by clicking on the link http://www.stata.com. Your window should look similar to figure 1.2.

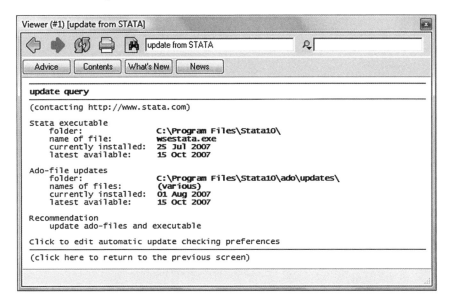

Figure 1.2. Viewer window after installing recommended updates

Look to see if you have the latest executable and ado-files. If not, follow the recommendation. In this case, click on update ado-files and executable. You are now told which ado-files were updated. This time the executable is updated, too (in most updates, only ado-files are updated). See figure 1.3.

(*Continued on next page*)

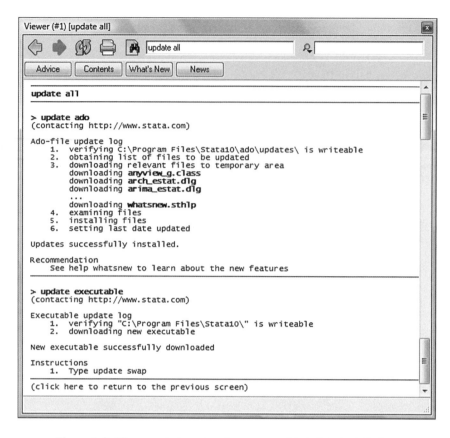

Figure 1.3. Viewer window showing successful update installation

IMPORTANT: If you download a new executable, you must install it before you can use it. Do that by typing the command `update swap` or by clicking on the `update swap` link. The screen flickers a bit—and then you should have the updated version of Stata. If the message `no; data in memory would be lost` is displayed, it means that you have a dataset loaded. You must first save your dataset and then `update swap`, or, if you do not want to save your data, you may enter the following commands in the Command window:

```
. clear
. update swap
```

After an update, you can see what was replaced and why by typing

```
. help whatsnew
```

Downloading the files for an update may take some time, so be patient. If you lose the connection during the update, no harm is done, and you can safely repeat the procedure.

If you have trouble updating, see the Stata web page http://www.stata.com/support/updates/ for some alternative solutions.

Updating regularly is a must!

Stata will ask you regularly if you want to check for updates. Accept the offer; it is easy — and important.

Where did Stata put the program files?

When installing, Stata typically creates the folders shown below. The main program (the executable) is installed in C:\Program Files\Stata10, whereas many commands are defined by ado-files (see section 17.3) to be installed in C:\Program Files\Stata10\ado\base. When updating, Stata installs new and revised ado-files in
C:\Program Files\Stata10\ado\updates.

Many ado-files have been written by creative users, not by Stata; see section 2.2 to learn how to locate them. Such files are installed in C:\ado\plus. You can store your own ado-files in C:\ado\personal. The main folders for the Stata program typically are

```
C:\
     ado
          personal            Your own creations (e.g., ado-files, profile.do)
          plus                Downloaded "unofficial" ado-files,
                                  e.g., user-written programs
     ...
     Program Files
          Stata10             The main program (executable)
               ado
                    base      Official ado-files as shipped with Stata
                    updates   Official ado-file updates
```

You can display these folders by typing the sysdir command:

```
. sysdir
    STATA:  C:\Program Files\Stata10\
  UPDATES:  C:\Program Files\Stata10\ado\updates\
     BASE:  C:\Program Files\Stata10\ado\base\
     SITE:  C:\Program Files\Stata10\ado\site\
     PLUS:  c:\ado\plus\
 PERSONAL:  c:\ado\personal\
 OLDPLACE:  c:\ado\
```

When you issue a command, Stata searches the currently active folder and these folders (called the *ado-path*) in the sequence shown until it finds a command with that name. If the command fails, Stata displays an error message.

1.2   Starting and exiting Stata

Starting Stata

There are several ways to start Stata; see [GSW] **2 Starting and exiting Stata**. In Windows, you can use one of the following methods:

- Select [Start] ▷ All Programs ▷ Stata.
- If you have a Stata desktop icon (see section 1.3), double-click on it.
- Open Explorer or My Computer, and double-click on a file with the extension .do or .dta.

But take care: any of these methods will open a new Stata session, even if one is already active, and you may end up with two or three Stata sessions running at the same time. This can be confusing and may cause problems with your log files (see section 1.6).

Exiting Stata

To stop Stata, you can do one of the following:

- Select File ▷ Exit.
- Click the [x] button in the upper-right corner of the screen.
- Type exit in the Command window.

If you have modified the data in memory without saving the modifications, you will be asked to choose Save or Don't save. If you make modifications intended to be permanent, make them with a do-file ending with a save command (see section 6.1), saving the modified dataset with a new name. If you have done that, Stata will not ask the question. If Stata asks you, it is likely that you made modifications not intended to be permanent, and the risk is that you overwrite good data with bad data if you respond Save.

You can avoid the above question by typing exit, clear in the Command window, and the current memory contents will not be saved.

1.3   Customizing Stata (Windows)

Creating a desktop shortcut icon

If a desktop shortcut icon was not created during installation, use Explorer or My Computer to locate the executable in C:\Program Files\Stata10. In Stata/IC for Windows, it is wstata.exe; in Stata/SE, it is wsestata.exe. Right-click on it and select Create Short-cut. This creates a shortcut icon that you can drag to the desktop.

Right-click on the new icon and select **Properties**. Select your personal main folder as the start folder. In this book's examples, it is `C:\docs` (see chapter 21 on Windows). Below you will find the reasons for this recommendation:

- You should put your own text, graphs, data files, and do-files in folders organized and named by subject, not by the program that created them; otherwise, you will end up confused.

- All of your own folders should be in subfolders under one personal main folder, e.g., `C:\docs`. The two advantages to this are that

  - You avoid mixing your own files with program files.
  - You can set up a consistent backup strategy (see section 18.9).

- Above all, do not put your own files in the `C:\Program Files\Stata10` folder (the Stata program folder).

1.4 Windows in Stata

[GSW] **4 The Stata user interface** gives a nice introduction to Stata's windows, including the use of the various buttons. Here I show how to define a rather simple and robust setup. The experienced user may want to experiment more. Start by selecting the factory settings for the layout of windows.

> Edit ▷ Preferences ▷ Manage Preferences ▷ Load Preferences ▷
> Factory Settings

Now adjust the size of the main Stata window. If you want it to fill the entire screen, click on the maximize ⬜ button (the middle button in the upper-right corner). Next adjust the other windows' sizes and locations with the mouse; it should look approximately like figure 1.4. When finished, make your choices the default by selecting

> Edit ▷ Preferences ▷ Manage Preferences ▷ Save Preferences

Save your preferences with a name, e.g., `myprefs`. If you somehow lost the settings, you can easily recreate them by selecting

> Edit ▷ Preferences ▷ Manage Preferences ▷ Load Preferences

If you right-click in a window, you get a list of options; one option is to change the font for that type of window; see [GSW] **18 Setting font and window preferences**. In the Results, Viewer, and Data windows, you can select a fixed-width font. The factory default is Lucida Console.

You can control the behavior of the windows by selecting

> Edit ▷ Preferences ▷ General Preferences...

A dialog box opens; select the Windowing tab to see checkboxes for a number of options. I suggest checking none of them, postponing any experiments for another day. Look at the possibilities in [GSW] **4 The Stata user interface**. And do not forget, when you are satisfied with a modified setup, save it by selecting

Edit ▷ Preferences ▷ Manage Preferences ▷ Save Preferences

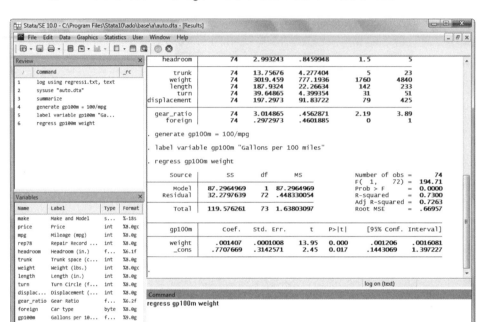

Figure 1.4. Recommended setup of the main windows in Stata

In the lower-left corner of the main Stata window, Stata displays the currently active folder, i.e., the folder where Stata expects files to be located and where files will be saved unless another folder is specified. In the Results window's lower-right corner, the current logging status (see section 1.6) is displayed.

Command window

In the Command window, you can enter single commands and execute them by pressing *Enter*.

While reading the rest of this chapter, you might benefit from having opened a dataset. In the Command window, give the command

```
. sysuse auto.dta
```

and see what happens. (auto is a dataset included in the installation. Automatically installed datasets are opened with the sysuse command rather than the use command.)

Results window

The Results window is the primary display of the output. You may print all or a selected part of the Results window. You can move around using the mouse or the keyboard; however, to make selections, you must use the mouse.

When the screen is full, it stops to let you read it, displaying more at the bottom of the screen. When you press the *Enter* key, the next line is displayed. If you press any other key, the next full screen is displayed. If you dislike the output interruptions created by more, you can type

```
. set more off
```

or, if you want this setting to be permanent, type

```
. set more off, permanently
```

To activate more again, type (do not type the brackets; they mean that permanently is optional)

```
. set more on [, permanently]
```

You can modify the colors displayed in the Results window, if you wish. I am red–green color-blind, and the default color scheme does not work well for me. It is especially important that error messages stand out. I also chose to underline links. To make these changes, select

Edit ▷ Preferences ▷ General Preferences...

which will bring up the General Preferences dialog box. In the Result Colors tab, select the color scheme "Custom 1". Click on a button to obtain the color palette, where you can change your color settings. For example, here are my color settings:

Result:	Light yellow
Standard:	Light yellow
Errors:	Strong yellow, bold
Input:	White
Link:	Light blue, underlined
Hilite:	White, bold
Background:	Black

The resulting dialog box for my settings is shown in figure 1.5.

(Continued on next page)

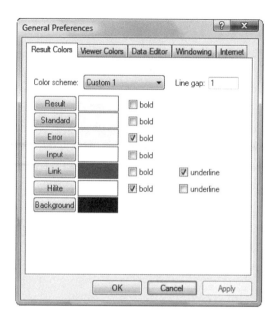

Figure 1.5. General Preferences dialog box

The initial buffer size for the Results window allows for only a few pages of output (32 KB). You may increase it, for example, to 200 KB by typing

```
. set scrollbufsize 200000
```

You must restart Stata for this setting to take effect.

Review window

The Review window displays the most recent commands. Click on a command in the Review window to paste it to the Command window, where you can edit and execute it. If you double-click a command in the Review window, it will be executed immediately. From the Command window, you can also scroll through past commands by using the *Page Up* and *Page Down* keys.

To copy commands to a do-file, click anywhere in the Review window. You can select one or more commands by using the mouse, or you can select all the commands by pressing *Ctrl+A*. Press *Ctrl+C* to copy the selected command to the Windows Clipboard. Next open a Do-file Editor window and paste the Review window contents by pressing *Ctrl+V*. An alternative route is to right-click in the Review window and use the contextual menu.

Variables window

The Variables window displays a list of the variables in memory and their labels. Insert a variable name in the Command window by clicking on it in the Variables window.

The Variables window initially displays four columns. By dragging in the top bar, I made the Label column wider, thus hiding the Type and Format columns, which I do not look at very often.

Viewer window

The main use of the Viewer window (figure 1.6) is to view help files (see section 2.2).

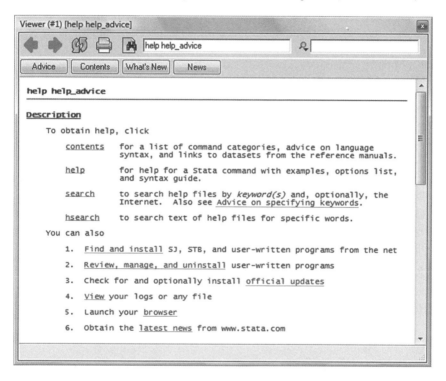

Figure 1.6. The Viewer window

The Viewer window can also be used to display and print output; see section 1.6. Read more in [GSW] **5 Using the Viewer**.

Open the Viewer window by clicking on the New Viewer button, ⬚. Try the various buttons and see what happens. If the text does not wrap correctly, click on the Refresh button,

.

You can have several Viewer windows open simultaneously. You can modify their appearance similarly to the Results window; I chose to underline links as in figure 1.6.

Data Editor/Browser

The Data Editor can be used in two modes: in *browse* mode, you can look at data without modifying them, while *edit* mode lets you modify and enter data.

The Data Editor looks like a spreadsheet, with variables as columns and observations as rows. String variables are displayed in red and value labels in blue. You may toggle between displaying codes and value labels by right-clicking somewhere in the Data Editor.

Click on the **Data Browser** button, ▨ , or type the `browse` command to see data in the Data Browser without the risk of making unintended changes. For example,

. `sysuse auto.dta`	Open dataset accompanying Stata
. `browse`	Show all variables, all observations
. `browse in 1/5`	Show all variables, first five observations
. `browse make weight length`	Show three variables, all observations
. `browse make in 23`	Show the variable make in the 23rd observation
. `browse mpg if foreign==1`	Show the variable mpg, foreign cars only

To open the Data Editor in edit mode, click on the **Data Editor** button, ▨ . You can now use the Data Editor to enter data; see [GSW] **8 Using the Data Editor**. There are, however, better ways to enter data; see some advice in section 6.2. You can also make changes and corrections to the data, but my general recommendation is to make corrections and other permanent modifications to the data with a do-file; see section 18.6.

When the Data Editor is open, you cannot do anything else in Stata. Close it to proceed.

Do-file Editor

The Do-file Editor is a standard text editor used for writing text files (typically do-files and ado-files). Open it by clicking on the **Do-file Editor** button, ▨ . The Do-file Editor has a special feature that you can use to execute all or a selection of the commands by clicking on the Do button, ▨ , or by pressing *Ctrl+D*. The **Run** button, ▨ , is rarely used. Read more in [GSW] **14 Using the Do-file Editor — automating Stata**.

You may check for balanced parentheses. Put the cursor inside a pair of parentheses and press *Ctrl+B*. Try it. It is easier to do than to explain.

Right-click anywhere in a Do-file Editor window to set your preferences, e.g., the font.

You can have several Do-file Editor windows open simultaneously, and in each window, you can have access to several do-files.

1.5   Issuing commands

Using the Command window

In the Command window, you can enter a command and execute it by pressing *Enter.* If the command fails, use *Page Up* to see it again and make modifications. You can also paste a previously used command to the Command window by clicking on the command in the Review window.

Using dialogs to generate commands

The dialogs let you generate complex commands without looking them up in the manuals or the online help. You may need to do some revising if you are not quite satisfied with the result.

There are two ways to activate a dialog. One is to use the menu system to find it. The dialog box for listing observations (the `list` command) is found by selecting

Data ▷ Describe data ▷ List data

If you know the command name, it is faster to open the dialog box by typing

. `db` *command*

A word in italics indicates that you should substitute something in place of that word. Here you would substitute the name of the command (e.g., `list`) for which you want to open a dialog box.

`list` is a simple and often-used command, and it is easier to enter it in the Command window, but for graphs and many analyses, the dialogs are a blessing. To understand the opportunities fully, you must, however, have some basic understanding of Stata's command syntax rules; see chapter 4. In section 11.10, I illustrate the use of a dialog to create a graph command.

Using do-files

A do-file is a series of commands to be executed in sequence. For any major task, this method is preferable to entering single commands because

- you make sure that the commands are executed in the sequence intended.
- if you discover an error, you can easily correct it and rerun the do-file.
- the do-file serves as documentation of what you did.

(*Continued on next page*)

A do-file is a plain-text (ASCII) file; it might look like the following:

```
——————————————— regress1.do ———————————————
* regress1.do
* Regression analysis of inverse mileage, with -rvfplot-.
sysuse auto.dta
generate gp100m = 100/mpg
label variable gp100m "Gallons per 100 miles"
summarize gp100m
regress gp100m weight
rvfplot, yline(0)
```

I always start a do-file with a comment stating the do-file's name (here * regress1.do. Stata interprets a line starting with * as a comment). This is useful so that you can identify the filename in a printout. Here I let the second comment line state the purpose of the do-file. The next six commands could have been given one by one in the Command window, but together they constitute an analysis, and keeping them together is extremely practical.

Use the Do-file Editor or another text editor to write your do-files.

Note: The last line in a do-file (and an ado-file) must end with a carriage return, or it will not work. The Do-file Editor automatically takes care of that, but if you use another text editor, you must include a carriage return.

The do command

Find and execute a do-file by selecting

     File ▷ Do...

or by typing the path and filename in the Command window after the do command:

    . do "C:\docs\proj1\regress1.do"

If C:\docs\proj1 is the current folder (look at the Stata screen's lower-left corner), you need only to type

    . do regress1.do

You can use the cd command (see section 6.1) to change the current folder

    . cd "C:\docs\proj1"

From the Do-file Editor, you can also execute the current do-file or a selected part of it by clicking on the Do button, [D] , or by pressing *Ctrl+D*. This method is easy but has the disadvantage that the do-file is not identified by name but rather by the name of a temporary file.

The Run button, ⬚ , corresponds to the `run` command. It executes the commands without displaying any output. I rarely use it.

1.6 Managing output

This section describes how to manage the output, primarily for printing. Find exercises about managing output in section 20.2.

The output log file

You can have Stata write a copy of the output you see in the Results window to an output log file; see [GSW] **17 Saving and printing results by using logs** and [U] **15 Printing and preserving output**. Activate an output log file by typing one of the following commands:

. `log using` *logfilename*, `replace`   Overwrite old log file
. `log using` *logfilename*, `append`   Append to existing log file

You can suspend logging by typing

. `log off`

and resume logging by typing

. `log on`

You can also stop logging by typing

. `log close`

The output log can be written in two formats: Stata Markup and Control Language (SMCL),[2] which can be displayed by the Viewer only, and plain ASCII text, which can be displayed by a text editor, a word processor, or the Viewer. Select the format by choosing a filename extension.

. `log using "C:\stata.smcl", replace`   SMCL format for display in the Viewer
. `log using "C:\stata.log", replace`   Text format for display in a text editor

You can see the current log status by typing

. `log`

The Log button, ⬚ , lets you open, close, and view the output log file. *Ctrl+L* has the same effect.

---

2. SMCL is a lot like HTML and is used for formatting help files and for formatting output displayed in the Viewer window.

If you installed the programs accompanying this book (see the book's web page, http://www.stata-press.com/books/ishr2.html), you can discard the current output log and open a new log with the same name by typing

```
. newlog
```

See section 17.5 if you want to know how `newlog` works.

Commands to be executed at program start: profile.do

To the inexperienced user, the easiest strategy is to have Stata open an output log file automatically at the start of the program. Some experienced users prefer to open a new output log file for each new major task, but my advice is to let Stata open a default output log file when you start the program.

If you have a `profile.do` file in the ado-path, the commands will be executed automatically each time you open Stata; see [GSW] **C.3 Executing commands every time Stata is started**. Let `profile.do` open an output log file (`stata.log` or `stata.smcl`) and a command log file (`cmdlog.txt`). Write your `profile.do` using Stata's Do-file Editor, and save it in the `C:\ado\personal` folder.[3] The simplest version looks like this:

```
─────────────────── C:\ado\personal\profile.do ───────────────────
* C:\ado\personal\profile.do
log using "C:\stata.log", replace        // open output log (text)
cmdlog using "C:\cmdlog.txt", append     // open command log
```

`log` opens Stata's output log file (`stata.log`) at the start of the session to receive the full output. The `replace` option overwrites output from the previous Stata session. If you want to take advantage of the SMCL formatting, the second line in `profile.do` should be

```
. log using "C:\stata.smcl", replace        Open output log ( SMCL)
```

I prefer the text format because it gives more freedom when handling the output. SMCL formatting requires that you inspect the output in the Viewer.

`cmdlog` opens Stata's command log file (`cmdlog.txt`) to receive the commands issued. The `append` option keeps the command log from previous sessions and allows you to examine and to reuse past commands. The command log file is described in section 1.7.

In section 17.5, you see a more elaborate `profile.do`. You can download it from the book's web site.

---

3. [GSW] **C.3 Executing commands every time Stata is started** recommends saving `profile.do` elsewhere. I stick to my recommendation; this folder is safer, and the commands in `profile.do` will be executed no matter how you start Stata.

Inspecting output in the Viewer window

If you let `profile.do` create the output log file `C:\stata.smcl`, you can open it in the Viewer by typing

```
. view "C:\stata.smcl"
```

You can also click on the **Log** button, , or press *Ctrl+L* to inspect the output log.

In the Viewer, you can select text (by using the mouse, not the keyboard) and print it. If the Viewer does not display the most recent output, click on the **Refresh** button, . You cannot edit the contents of the Viewer.

Inspecting output in a text editor

You can use any text editor to examine output. Compared with using the Viewer, the advantage of using a text editor is that you can remove errors and mistakes before printing and add comments to the output, so you have more freedom when working with the output. If you want to use a text editor to inspect output, let `profile.do` create `C:\stata.log` (text format); see above.

You can find a thorough assessment of several text editors in an FAQ by Cox (2005) by typing

```
. findit text editors
```

My favorite text editor is NoteTab Light, which you can download for free. You can find a short description and a link to its web site at the author's web site; see *Other supplementary materials provided by the author* at http://www.stata-press.com/books/ishr2.html. A major advantage of this text editor is that you have access to several files simultaneously. Each file has its own tab, hence the name. Section 17.5 shows the `nlog` command as an example of how you can use a third-party text editor — in this case, NoteTab Light — to inspect output. Find `nlog.ado` at this book's web site http://www.stata-press.com/books/ishr2.html.

Copying output to a word-processor document

From the Results window, the Viewer window, or a text editor, you can copy and paste a highlighted part of the output to a word-processor document. To align the text correctly, you must select a monospaced font in the word processor, e.g., Lucida Console 9 pt.

For many tables, you can obtain a more sophisticated result. You can copy results directly to a word-processor document as an HTML table, or you can use Microsoft Excel (or another spreadsheet program) as an intermediary agent. This method works best if the output is arranged in columns.

To copy results as an HTML table, do the following:

1. Highlight the table in the Results window. Right-click the mouse and select Copy Table as HTML.

2. Paste the table into your word-processor document. Once it is there, you should be able to right-click on it to format the cells.

To copy results by using a spreadsheet program, do the following:

1. Highlight the table in the Results window. Right-click the mouse and select Copy Table.

2. Paste the table (*Ctrl+V*) into your spreadsheet program. Format the table if needed, e.g., by adjusting the number of decimals (you will need to use the program's formatting tools).

3. Copy and paste the table from the spreadsheet to your word-processor document.

Decimal periods and commas

To copy output correctly, you must set both Windows and Stata to display decimals as periods or to display decimals as commas. To display commas in Stata, type set dp comma. To return to the default decimal periods, type set dp period. This setting affects only how values are displayed.

Stata commands always use decimal periods, and Stata cannot read or write ASCII data with decimal commas, regardless of the dp setting and the Windows settings (see section 6.3), so you should use decimal periods consistently. This is the default in Stata. In Windows, you can change the setting by selecting

[Start] ▷ Control Panel ▷ Regional and Language Options

Here you can choose a country that uses decimal periods.

If you are creating a graph and want axis labels with decimal commas, type set dp comma.

1.7   Reusing commands

As shown in section 1.4, the Review window displays the most recent commands issued. Click on a command to paste it to the Command window. To copy all the commands to a do-file, click inside the Review window and press *Ctrl+A* to highlight all commands and *Ctrl+C* to copy them to the Windows Clipboard. Next open a Do-file Editor window and paste the text with *Ctrl+V*. The do-file will probably need some editing.

You can have Stata copy all future commands within the current session to a command log file by typing

> . cmdlog using *cmdlogfilename* $\left[\,,\ \texttt{append}\,|\,\texttt{replace}\,\right]$

The command log is always plain text. If you, as I suggested in section 1.6, had profile.do generate a command log file (C:\cmdlog.txt), you can inspect it in the Do-file Editor. You can also copy and paste a group of commands to a new window, edit them, and save a revised do-file. Because we set the command log file to be cumulative (the `append` option), you can even access commands from previous sessions. Using a log this way is a good alternative to copying the Review window contents to the Do-file Editor.

An extended `profile.do`, shown in section 17.5, adds a time stamp to the cumulative command log when a new session starts to help you find past commands.

2 Getting help—and more

2.1 The manuals

For beginners, this book and the *Getting Started* manual might suffice, but this book does not replace the manuals. The manuals have much more detail and documentation than could be written in this book. [GSW], [U], [D], etc., refer to the official manuals:

[GS]   *Getting Started* gives an overview of Stata's main features. [GSW] is for the Windows version of Stata. There are similar introductions to the Unix and Macintosh versions as well.

[U]   *User's Guide* gives a systematic description of Stata.

[D]   *Data Management Reference Manual* includes commands for reading and saving files, making calculations, and modifying the data structure.

[R]   *Base Reference Manual* (three volumes) includes all general commands, except those in [D].

[ST]   *Survival Analysis and Epidemiological Tables Reference Manual* includes descriptive procedures, survival regression models, and procedures for the analysis of epidemiological tables.

[G]   *Graphics Reference Manual* includes information about Stata's graphics.

[I]   *Quick Reference and Index Manual* includes brief descriptions of Stata procedures and an index.

There are more manuals than these; see more about manuals and other useful books in chapter 19.

2.2 Online help

Keeping your Stata updated will update your online help, too. To read more about the online help, see [GSW] **6 Getting help** and [U] **4 Stata's online help and search facilities**. See also [R] **net** and [R] **search**.

help

The help command displays information in the Viewer window. You can also type help at the Viewer command line.

If you know a command name (e.g., tabstat), you can display a help file (tabstat.sthlp) by typing help *command*, for example,

. **help tabstat**

You can get the same result by clicking on

Help ▷ Stata Command...

and typing tabstat.

The help file is displayed in the Viewer window, and from here you can print it. You can also use the links included; try it. For more information on the contents and interpretation of syntax diagrams and online help, see section 4.2.

You can also find help for functions, for example, the exp() (exponential) function:

. **help exp()**

help displays information stored on your computer, but you can also find help on the Internet.

Using the menus and dialogs

If you are searching for a command, a good strategy is to use the menus and dialogs. Suppose that you want to find out about Stata's facilities concerning nonparametric statistics.

Statistics ▷ Summaries, tables, and tests ▷ Nonparametric tests of hypotheses

This sequence displays a menu with (currently) 11 tests. If you select a test, for example, Kruskal–Wallis rank test, Stata opens a dialog. Click on the ❓ button in the dialog's lower-left corner to see the online help for the kwallis command.

search

You can find information about a command even if you do not know the command name.

For example, you can get information about nonparametric tests by typing

. **search nonparametric**

You can get the same result by clicking on

Help ▷ Search...

and typing nonparametric.

This search list refers to several official Stata entries, including

- Help files on your computer for several Stata commands
- FAQs (see section 2.3)
- Papers and programs published in the *Stata Journal* (SJ) and its predecessor, the *Stata Technical Bulletin* (STB). Note that you have free access to the STB at http://www.stata.com/bookstore/stbj.html. For the SJ, visit http://www.stata-journal.com/archives.html to see abstracts from the newer issues and the full text from issues more than three years old.

The Help ▷ Search... dialog also lets you search outside the official Stata; this dialog corresponds to the commands

```
. search nonparametric, net    Search official and unofficial web sites
. search nonparametric, all    Search your computer and all web sites
```

Unofficial web sites include several commands (ado-files) and papers generated by creative users. The largest such site is Statistical Software Components (SSC) at Boston College. Read more in [R] **ssc** or

```
. help ssc
```

The number of unofficial ado-files available may seem overwhelming, but I often find what I am looking for. One problem with unofficial programs is that there is no formal quality control. Errors do occur, even in the official programs, but Stata has formal procedures to ensure corrections once an error has been detected. To check for updates to unofficial commands you have installed on your computer, type

```
. adoupdate
```

findit

An easy alternative to search *search_term*, all is the findit command:

```
. findit nonparametric
```

Say that you are looking for a command that estimates sensitivity, specificity, and predictive values for a binary diagnostic test. You will want to include keywords that are likely to identify all relevant commands (a sensitivity issue) without pointing to too many irrelevant commands (the specificity problem). I chose

```
. findit sensitivity specificity
```

and found, among other things,

```
SJ-4-4  sbe36_2 . . . . . . . . . . . . . . . . . . . Software update for diagt
        (help diagt if installed) . . . . . . . . . P. T. Seed and A. Tobias
        Q4/04   SJ 4(4):490
        new options added to diagt
```

Currently, no official Stata command does what we want, but the unofficial command `diagt` seems to. Information on this procedure was published in the SJ, volume 4, number 4. Click on the link `sbe36_2` to obtain

---

```
package sbe36_2 from http://www.stata-journal.com/software/sj4-4
```

```
TITLE
      SJ4-4 sbe36_2.  Summary statistics for diagnostic tests

DESCRIPTION/AUTHOR(S)
      Summary statistics for diagnostic tests
      by Paul T. Seed, King's College London, UK
         Aurelio Tobias, Universidad Carlos III de Madrid, Spain
      Support:  paul.seed@kcl.ac.uk, atobias@wanadoo.es
      After installation, type help diagt and diagti

INSTALLATION FILES                          (click here to install)
      sbe36_2/diagt.ado
      sbe36_2/diagt.hlp
      sbe36_2/diagti.ado
      sbe36_2/diagti.hlp
```

```
(click here to return to the previous screen)
```

Now click on the link `click here to install`. Read the help file. The use of the `diagt` command is illustrated in section 15.3. Unofficial programs are automatically installed in `C:\ado\plus`.

2.3   Other resources

For an overview of available resources, see [U] **3 Resources for learning and using Stata**.

Stata NetCourses

Stata offers NetCourses to newcomers and advanced users. Read more about NetCourses at http://www.stata.com/netcourse.

FAQs

Stata's web site includes a lot of advice on various topics, including several FAQs. You can find these FAQs at http://www.stata.com/support/faqs/. You can look for information by using the structured list of contents, or you can perform a keyword search.

Say that you are uncertain about Stata's handling of missing values and want to see if there is an FAQ on the subject. Open http://www.stata.com/support/faqs/, and type `missing values` in the search field. From the articles listed, you may find this one promising: *Why is x > 1000 true when x contains missing value?* You would be led to the same FAQ (among many other items) if you typed

```
. findit missing values
```

Statalist

Statalist is a users' forum for exchange of questions, answers, advice, and ideas:

```
. help statalist
```

Stata technical support

You can email Stata and ask for help. You should, however, try to help yourself first by looking up the relevant information in the online help and the manuals. You can find good advice before emailing by typing

```
. search technical support
```

If you believe you have found an error, then by all means write to technical support. You may be right, but even if you are not, you will get a swift and informative answer. If possible, include a small dataset and a do-file demonstrating the problem.

Asking a more experienced user

The same considerations as above apply. Assuming that the more experienced user really wants to help you, consider what information the user will need. If you do not understand why something does not work, include output with commands and error messages.

2.4 Errors and error messages

Stata's short error messages include a code, e.g., r(131). The code is a link, which you can click on to get more information about the error. Designing useful error messages, however, is complicated, and Stata cannot always guess your intent, so you may not always find the error message to be helpful. The following sections discuss frequent errors and the corresponding error messages.

Stata is case sensitive

Remember that Stata is case sensitive; this applies both to Stata commands and to variables. Try typing

```
. List
unrecognized command:  List
r(199);
```

Stata told you that it did not recognize the List command. Click on the r(199) link to get more details:

```
[P]     error . . . . . . . . . . . . . . . . . . . . . . . . . Return code 199
        unrecognized command;
        Stata failed to recognize the command, program, or ado-file name,
        probably because of a typographical or abbreviation error.
```

The details are not informative, but you probably wanted to use the list command, which begins with a lowercase letter.

The equal-sign in relational expressions (==)

Remember the difference between the assignment equal-sign (=) and the relational equal-sign (==); see section 4.4.

```
. summarize if foreign = 1
invalid syntax
r(198);
```

To get more information, click on the r(198) link. It is not informative either. The actual error was that you used the single equal-sign in a relational expression, but it should have been

```
. summarize if foreign == 1
```

Commas and options

Misplacing the comma preceding options is a frequent beginner's error (experienced users do it, too):

```
. summarize, if foreign == 1
option if not allowed
r(198);
```

Stata interprets everything after a comma as an option. summarize has no if option. You probably wanted to use the if qualifier, which must be placed before any comma (see section 4.4), so the command should have been

```
. summarize if foreign == 1
```

Forgetting the comma is common, too:

```
. ttest price by(foreign)
time-series operators not allowed
r(101);
```

This error message was not helpful. You really did not do anything that should make Stata think of time-series analysis. However, by() is an option of ttest, so it should be preceded by a comma, and the command should have been

```
. ttest price, by(foreign)
```

Space between option names and arguments

There is no space between an option name and a subsequent parenthesis. Stata often forgives a space, but not always. The error message may be confusing:

```
. scatter mpg weight, xtitle ("Weight")
"Weight invalid name
r(198);
. scatter mpg weight, xtitle (Weight)
option xtitle() not allowed
r(198);
```

In both cases, there was an inappropriate space between xtitle and the parenthesis containing the argument. Both commands below are correct:

```
. scatter mpg weight, xtitle("Weight")
. scatter mpg weight, xtitle(Weight)
```

Such errors may be difficult to identify, especially in complex graph commands.

Stata does, however, forgive spaces around operators, such as == or >=. Thus foreign==1 and foreign == 1 are the same thing to Stata.

3 Stata file types and names

Stata works with several types of files. The most important types of files are shown below. The filename extension shows the file type, both to the user and to the operating system:

```
. use alpha.dta        Open Stata dataset
. do alpha.do          Execute Stata do-file
```

Often Stata allows you to omit the filename extension:

```
. use alpha            Open Stata dataset
. do alpha             Execute Stata do-file
```

However, including the filename extension makes the command more transparent, and I will do that throughout this book. This advice is consistent with my advice to let Windows display filename extensions; see chapter 21. Use quotation marks around a filename if it includes spaces.

.dta files: Stata data

The extension for a Stata dataset is .dta. Stata datasets can be interpreted only by Stata and by programs specifically designed to read Stata datasets, such as Stat/Transfer.

.do files: command files

A do-file with the extension .do is a group of commands to be executed in sequence. Do-files are in plain-text (ASCII) format and can be edited and displayed by any text editor, such as Stata's Do-file Editor.

You can issue single commands in the Command window, but if you are doing anything substantial, you should use a do-file; see section 1.5.

.ado files: programs

An ado-file with the extension .ado is a program. Ado-files are in plain-text format. For more information, see section 17.3.

.sthlp files: Stata help

Stata's online documentation is stored in .sthlp files, written in SMCL format, which is somewhat like HTML. SMCL-formatted files can be displayed in the Viewer window. Prior to Stata 10, these files had the extension .hlp and were sometimes confused with Windows' help files. Old Stata .hlp files still work.

If you look in the Stata folders, you will also see .ihlp files, which contain help that can be reused in several help files.

.gph files: graphs

Stata graphs can be saved as .gph files; see section 11.9.

.txt files: plain ASCII format

A plain-text file simply includes lines of text (the text may also be numbers). The Stata manuals give such files the extension .raw, whereas most other Windows applications, by default, use the extension .txt. In this book, I will use the extension .txt.

.scheme: settings for graphs

To control the appearance of graphs, use the extension .scheme; see section 11.4.

There are more file types than the ones listed in this chapter. For an overview, see [U] **11.6 File-naming conventions**.

4 Command syntax

4.1 General syntax rules

Stata's command syntax rules are described in detail in [U] **11 Language syntax**.

Stata is case sensitive, and almost all Stata commands are lowercase. `list` is a valid command, but `List` is not. Variable names may include lowercase and uppercase letters, but `sex` and `Sex` are two different variable names. Throughout this book, I use lowercase variable names.

Variable names can have 1–32 characters, but Stata often abbreviates long variable names in output, so I recommend using 10 characters at most. The letters a–z, the numbers 0–9, and _ (underscore) are valid characters. Non-English characters like ü, ø, è, and ž are not accepted or at least not safe. Names must start with a letter (or an underscore, but this is strongly discouraged because many Stata-generated temporary variables start with an underscore). The following are valid variable names:

```
a q17 q_17 pregnant sex
```

4.2 Syntax diagrams

A syntax diagram is a formal description of the elements in a Stata command. The notation used is described in [R] **intro** (in the beginning of the first volume).

The general syntax of typical Stata commands can be written like this:

$$\big[\,prefix\!:\,\big]\ command\ \big[\,varlist\,\big]\ \big[\,if\,\big]\ \big[\,in\,\big]\ \big[\,weight\,\big]\ \big[\,,\ options\,\big]$$

For example, the syntax for `summarize` is

$$\underline{\texttt{su}}\texttt{mmarize}\ \left[\textit{varlist}\right]\ \left[\textit{if}\right]\ \left[\textit{in}\right]\ \left[\textit{weight}\right]\ \left[\texttt{,}\ \textit{options}\right]$$

options	description
Main	
<u>d</u>etail	display additional statistics
<u>mea</u>nonly	suppress the display; calculate only the mean; programmer's option
<u>f</u>ormat	use variable's display format
<u>s</u>eparator(*#*)	draw separator line after every # variables; default is `separator(5)`

varlist may contain time-series operators; see [U] **11.4.3 Time-series varlists**.
by is allowed; see [D] **by**.
`aweights`, `fweights`, and `iweights` are allowed. However, `iweights` may not be used
   with the `detail` option; see [U] **11.1.6 weight**.

Thin square brackets, [ ], mean that the item is optional, so the only mandatory part of the `summarize` syntax is the command name itself. Square brackets may also be part of the syntax, in which case they are shown in the typewriter font, as in

    tab2 case ctrl [fweight=pop]

Curly brackets, { }, mean that you must specify one of the options, but not both options, as in

$$\texttt{numlabel}\ \left[\textit{lblname-list}\right]\texttt{,}\ \left\{\underline{\texttt{a}}\texttt{dd}\,|\,\underline{\texttt{r}}\texttt{emove}\right\}$$

Here you must specify either `add` or `remove`.

Command and option names can be abbreviated; underlining shows the minimum abbreviation. I use few abbreviations because, although they make commands faster to write, they are difficult to read.

Table 4.1 shows some example `summarize` commands

Table 4.1. Example `summarize` commands

prefix	command	varlist	qualifiers/weights	options	comments
	`summarize`	`_all`			`_all`: all variables
	`summarize`				All variables
	`sum`				Abbreviated
	`summarize`	`sex age`			Two variables
	`summarize`	`sex-weight`			Variable range
	`summarize`	`pro*`			All variables starting with `pro`
	`summarize`	`*ro*`			All variables containing `ro`
	`summarize`	`??ro?`			5-letter variables with `ro` as 3rd and 4th characters
	`summarize`	`age`	`if sex==1`		Males only
	`summarize`	`bmi`	`in 1/10`		First 10 observations
	`summarize`	`bmi`	`[fweight=n]`		Weighted observations
`by sex:`	`sort` `summarize`	`sex` `bmi`			Separate table for each `sex`; data must be sorted first
	`summarize`	`bmi`		`, detail`	Option: `detail`

Figure 4.1 is the online help for `summarize`, which is displayed in the Viewer window by typing

`. help summarize`

(*Continued on next page*)

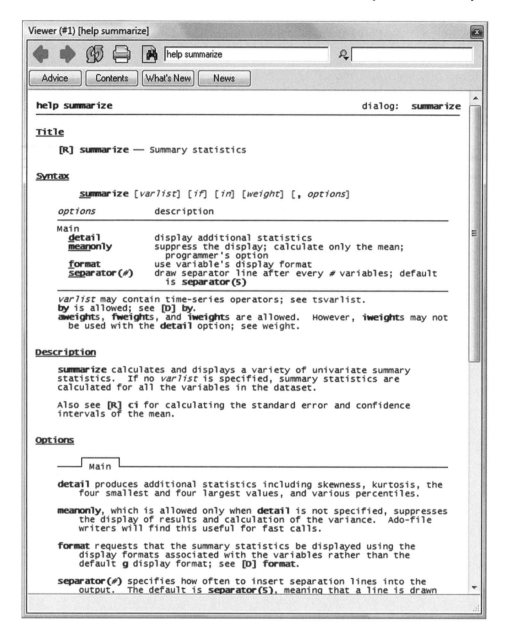

Figure 4.1. Online help for summarize

The help description includes several links to related commands and other information. Compared with the information in the *Base Reference Manual*, the online help is brief. The manuals typically include more elaborate examples, a description of statistical methods, and references.

4.3 Lists of variables and numbers

Variable lists

A variable list (*varlist*) defines one or more variables to be processed; see [U] **11.1.1 varlist**. Here are some examples:

(nothing)	Sometimes means the same as _all
_all	All variables in the dataset
sex age pregnant	Three variables
pregnant sex-weight	pregnant and the consecutive variables from sex to weight
pro*	All variables starting with pro
ro	All variables containing ro
??ro?	5-letter variables with ro as third and fourth characters

When generating new variables, you can refer to the 17 variables q1, q2, ..., q17 as q1-q17. When referring to the existing variables q1-q17, you will get q1, q17, and the variables that come between them in the dataset, but they are not necessarily the 15 variables q2, q3, ..., q16. summarize and describe are useful commands to see the ordering of variables in the dataset.

In commands that have a dependent variable, it is listed first in the variable list:

. oneway bmi sex	bmi is the dependent variable
. regress bmi sex age	bmi is the dependent variable
. scatter weight height	Scatterplot, weight is the y-axis
. tab2 expos case	The first variable defines the rows

Numeric lists

A numeric list (*numlist*) is a list of numbers with some shorthand possibilities (see [U] **11.1.8 numlist**):

1(3)11	means	1 4 7 10
1(1)4 4.5(0.5)6	means	1 2 3 4 4.5 5 5.5 6
4 3 2 7(-1)1	means	4 3 2 7 6 5 4 3 2 1
1/5	means	1 2 3 4 5
4/2 7/1	means	4 3 2 7 6 5 4 3 2 1

Numeric lists have many uses; for example, they can

- Display person–time and incidence rates every 0.5 years, up to 5 years:

    `. stptime, at(0(0.5)5) by(drug)`
- Show a graph with y-axis labels at 0 10 20 30 40:

    `. scatter mpg weight, ylabel(0(10)40)`
- Generate age groups 0–4, 5–14, 15–24, ..., 75–84, 85+:

    `. egen agegrp = cut(age), at(0 5(10)85 200)`

Numeric ranges

Numeric lists should not be confused with numeric ranges. The following are ranges:

```
. list in 1/10
. recode age (0/24=1)(25/44=2)(45/max=3), generate(agegr)
```

4.4   Qualifiers

Qualifiers are common to many commands, while most options are specific to one or a few commands.

The if qualifier

The `if` qualifier is used with logical expressions to select the observations to which a command applies; see [U] **11.1.3 if exp**. Here are a few examples:

`. summarize age if sex == 1`	Males only
`. summarize age if sex != 1`	Males excluded
`. list id age if age <= 25`	Young only
`. replace npreg=. if sex == 1`	Males: npreg missing
`. list sex age weight if sex == 1 & age <= 25`	Young males only
`. keep if sex == 1 | age <= 25`	Males or young
`. keep if !(sex == 1 | age <= 25)`	All others

Two types of operators are used in logical expressions (see table 4.2); see [U] **13.2 Operators**.

Table 4.2. Operators in logical expressions

Relational operators		Logical operators	
>	Greater than	!	Not
<	Less than	~	Not
>=	Greater than or equal to	&	And
<=	Less than or equal to	|	Or
==	Equal		
!=	Not equal		
~=	Not equal		

The double equal-sign, "==", in relational expressions has a meaning different from that of the assignment equal-sign, as in

```
. generate bmi = weight/(height^2)
```

Logical expressions are evaluated to true or false. A value of 0 means false, and any other value, including missing values, means true. Technically, missing values are large positive numbers and are evaluated as such in logical expressions; see [U] **12.2.1 Missing values**. This behavior leads to the following warning:

Warning: Missing values in logical expressions

The following command initially surprised me by listing all whose ages were greater than 65 *and* those with a missing age:

```
. list id age if age > 65
```

Technically, a missing value is larger than any valid number, which means that the expression age > 65 is true if age is missing. To exclude the missing values, type

```
. list id age if age > 65 & age < .
```

or

```
. list id age if age > 65 & !missing(age)
```

To list the missing values only, including user-defined missing values, type

```
. list id age if age >= .
```

or

```
. list id age if missing(age)
```

See [U] **12.2.1 Missing values** for more information.

In the `auto.dta` dataset, the variable `foreign` takes the values 0 and 1. You may see a construct like

```
. keep if foreign
```

`foreign` can be evaluated as a logical expression, being false if `foreign` is 0 and true otherwise. I find this method a bit dangerous because any observations with `foreign` missing would be included, too, and that might not be what you intended.

With complex logical expressions, use parentheses to control the order of evaluation:

```
. anycommand if ((sex==1 & weight>90) | (sex==2 & weight>80))
> & weight<.
```

Omitting the parentheses might give a different selection, but the outcome may be difficult to predict. Use parentheses to make the syntax transparent to yourself; then it will work correctly. Another way to handle complex selections is to generate a help variable (`heavy`).

`. generate heavy=0`	Initialize help variable
`. replace heavy=1 if sex==1 & weight>90`	Include males > 90 kg
`. replace heavy=1 if sex==2 & weight>80`	Include females > 80 kg
`. replace heavy=. if weight>=.`	Don't include if `weight` is missing
`. anycommand if heavy==1`	These are the heavy ones

The in qualifier

The `in` qualifier is used to select the observations to which a command applies; see [U] **11.1.4 in range**. It is especially useful for listing or displaying a subset of observations. Below are three examples:

`. list sex age weight in 23`	23rd observation
`. list in 1/10`	All variables; observations 1–10
`. browse sex-weight in -5/-1`	See last 5 observations in the Data Browser

The last observation is identified by –1, and –5/–1 means the last 5 observations.

4.5   Weights

Weighting observations

Weights can be used to "multiply" observations when the input is tabular; see [U] **11.1.6 weight**. Suppose that you see the following table in a paper and want to analyze it further:

	Cases	Controls
Exposed	21	30
Unexposed	23	100
Total	44	130

The input command (see section 6.2) lets you enter the tabular data directly:

```
. input expos case pop
  1 1 21
  1 0 30
  0 1 23
  0 0 100
  end
```

Now you can analyze the data by weighting with pop:

```
. tab2 expos case [fweight=pop], chi2
. cc expos case [fweight=pop]
```

The square brackets around the weight expression are in the typewriter font and are part of the syntax. Here they do not mean "optional".

fweight indicates frequency weighting. For information about other types of weighting, see [U] **20.17 Weighted estimation**. Instead of weighting the analysis, you could expand the dataset; see section 9.6.

4.6 Options

Options are specific to a command, and you must look in the manuals or the online help to see the options that are available; see [U] **11.1.7 options**. Options come last in the command, and they are preceded by a comma. Usually, there is only one comma per command, but complex graph commands may include more than one; see chapter 11.

The nolabel option is common to many commands. If value labels have been assigned to a variable, Stata usually displays the value label rather than the code in tables and listings. The nolabel option lets you see the code instead of the label:

```
. sysuse auto.dta, clear
(1978 Automobile Data)

. tab1 foreign

-> tabulation of foreign
```

Car type	Freq.	Percent	Cum.
Domestic	52	70.27	70.27
Foreign	22	29.73	100.00
Total	74	100.00	

```
. tab1 foreign, nolabel
-> tabulation of foreign
```

Car type	Freq.	Percent	Cum.
0	52	70.27	70.27
1	22	29.73	100.00
Total	74	100.00	

The same option applies to browsing (looking at the Data window):

```
. browse displacement-foreign in 1/2            Display any labels
. browse displacement-foreign in 1/2, nolabel   Display codes
```

In the Data window, you can toggle between codes and value labels (blue text) by right-clicking somewhere in the Data window.

The missing option is also common to many commands. It means that missing codes are included in tabulations, etc., like any other category.

Another common option is level(). It is used to specify confidence levels other than the default 95%. You could specify 90% confidence intervals by typing

```
. regress mpg weight, level(90)
```

4.7   Prefixes

Only the by *varlist*: prefix is shown here, but there are others, e.g., xi: (see section 13.1).

The by varlist: prefix

See [U] **11.5 by varlist: construct**. The by *varlist*: prefix makes a command perform calculations or display results for strata of the data. Data must be sorted by the stratification variables. The following commands lead to two summarize tables, one for each sex:

```
. sort sex
. by sex: summarize age height weight
```

You can produce the same results with a single command:

```
. bysort sex: summarize age height weight
```

4.8   Other syntax elements

Text strings with quotes

Stata requires double quotes around text strings that contain embedded blank spaces or commas:

```
. label define sex  1 male  2 female  9 "sex unknown"
```

You need not use quotes around filenames and file paths, such as

```
. save alpha1.dta
```

unless they include a blank space:

```
. save "alpha 1.dta"
```

Comments

See [U] **16.1.2 Comments and blank lines in do-files**. The following are interpreted as comments, so you can include short explanations in do-files and ado-files:

- Lines beginning with ∗
- Text surrounded by /∗ and ∗/
- Text following // (// must be preceded by a space if they are not the first characters on the line)

Comments make your do-files more readable; Stata does not care what you write:

```
* C:\ado\personal\profile.do executes when opening Stata

summarize bmi, detail            // Body mass index
```

The above applies to do-files and ado-files. In the Command window, you may enter a comment with ∗, but not with // or /∗...∗/.

Long lines in do-files and ado-files

See [U] **16.1.3 Long lines in do-files**. In do-files and ado-files, a command, by default, ends when the line ends (carriage return), and no special delimiter terminates commands. However, command lines in do-files and ado-files should be no longer than 80 characters for readability on most screens. This problem is solved by typing /// to indicate that the following line is a continuation. /// must be preceded by a space.

```
infix str10 cprstr 1-10 bday 1-2 bmon 3-4 byear 5-6    ///
     control 7-10 using datefile.txt
```

Another option is to define ; (the semicolon) as the future command delimiter:

```
#delimit ;               // Semicolon delimits future commands

infix str10 cprstr 1-10 bday 1-2 bmon 3-4 byear 5-6
     control 7-10 using "datefile.txt";
tab1 byear;

#delimit cr              // Back to normal: Carriage return delimiter
```

Text enclosed by /* and */ is also interpreted as a comment. It can then be used to "comment out" a carriage return:

```
infix str10 cprstr 1-10 bday 1-2 bmon 3-4 byear 5-6     /*
    */ control 7-10 using "datefile.txt"
```

Note: The above does not apply to commands entered in the Command window. Here you just continue writing the command until you are finished and then press *Enter*. In the Command window, the // comment characters and the /// continuation characters are not allowed, but you may use * to insert a comment.

In output, a long command entered in the Command window will be displayed like this:

```
. infix str10 cprstr 1-10 bday 1-2 bmon 3-4 byear 5-6 control 7-10
> using "datefile.txt"
```

The > will precede any line after the first, and you should not type it.

Abbreviating command, option, and variable names

See [U] **11.2 Abbreviation rules**. In commands, you can abbreviate variable names to the minimum number of characters that unambiguously identify the variable. As shown in section 4.2, you can also abbreviate command and option names. This means that the command

```
. summarize age if sex==1, detail
```

can be abbreviated to

```
. su a if s==1, d
```

unless there are other variables in the dataset starting with a or s.

I rarely use abbreviations. It is more important that the command be easy to read than easy to write, and with abbreviations, the risk of mistakes is rather high. You may develop your private habits, but try to make the syntax readable when communicating with others (please!). If you look at or participate in the exchanges at Statalist (see section 2.3), you might meet syntax like

```
. qui su
```

This might make no sense whatsoever to you. Fortunately, the help system understands the abbreviations, so typing

```
. help qui
```

tells you that the command is quietly. From here it is easy; the full command is

```
. quietly summarize
```

4.9 Version control

New commands and features are introduced with every new version of Stata. For an overview of changes from version 9 to version 10, read [U] **1.3 What's new** or type the command

```
. help whatsnew9to10
```

Sometimes introducing new features leads to modification of the syntax of an existing command, and syntax that worked in version 9 may not work in version 10. This can be an inconvenience, but Stata preserves the old meanings of commands via version control.

An example: With Stata 10, the properties of date variables changed so that date information could be combined with time-of-day information; see section 5.5. This made it necessary to change the syntax for some functions. The date() function extracts information from a text string. In version 10, a day-month-year sequence of date elements is defined by the "DMY" specification. This is how date1 in the example below is generated.

The command attempting to generate date2 uses version 9 syntax. Here the sequence definition was lowercase, "dmy". The result becomes missing because Stata 10 does not understand this syntax. However, with a version 9: prefix, the command is parsed using version 9 rules, and date3 is generated correctly.

With the version command, you can specify which version is used to parse the commands that follow version; here version 9.2 governs the command generating date4. After that command, control is returned to version 10.

```
. set obs 1
obs was 0, now 1
. generate strdate = "17.1.2001"
. generate date1 = date(strdate,"DMY")
. generate date2 = date(strdate,"dmy")
 (1 missing value generated)
. version 9: gen date3 = date(strdate,"dmy")
. version
version 10.0
. version 9.2
. generate date4 = date(strdate,"dmy")
. version 10
. format date1 date2 date3 date4 %td
. list
```

	strdate	date1	date2	date3	date4
1.	17.1.2001	17jan2001	.	17jan2001	17jan2001

5 Variables

A Stata dataset is rectangular. Here is an example with five observations and four variables:

	obsno	age	height	weight
			Variables	
	1	27	178	74
	2	54	166	67
Observations	3	63	173	85
	4	36	182	81
	5	57	165	90

This corresponds to what you see in Stata's Data window when you issue a `browse` command.

5.1 Types of variables

Stata has two main types of variables: numeric and string. String variables are described in section 5.6. Read more about variable types in [U] **12 Data** and [D] **data types**.

Date and time variables are a special variety of numeric variables; see section 5.5.

For most purposes, numeric variables are more useful than string variables, and some analyses do not work with string variables. Sections 5.2–5.4 deal with numeric variables only. You might decide to postpone reading sections 5.5 and 5.6 until you feel the need.

5.2 Numeric formats

See [U] **12.5.1 Numeric formats** and [D] **format**. Format means display format (see table 5.1). A format specification does not affect the values in the dataset but only the way they are displayed in the output. You can see the formats applied to variables in a dataset by typing

    . describe [varlist]

Table 5.1. Numeric display formats

Format	Formula	Example	$\sqrt{2}$	1,000	10,000,000
General	*%w.dg*	%9.0g	1.414214	1000	1.00e+07
Fixed	*%w.df*	%9.0f	1	1000	10000000
		%9.2f	1.41	1000.00	1.00e+07
		%09.2f	000001.41	001000.00	1.00e+07
Exponential	*%w.de*	%10.3e	1.414e+00	1.000e+03	1.000e+07

w: The total width, including period and decimals
d: Number of decimals

The default is the g (general) format, displaying values with reasonable precision. Usually, you need not bother with numeric formats, but you can specify a fixed (f) format, e.g.,

```
. format usd eur %10.2f
. format jpy %10.0fc
. list in 1/3, clean
          usd        eur        jpy
  1.    1645.82    1362.40    192,308
  2.   22628.54   18731.74  2,644,058
  3.   12693.05   10507.22  1,483,135
```

For jpy, the c in the format specification means to display commas as thousands delimiters.

set dp comma displays decimal commas, but you must still use decimal periods in commands. Displaying decimal commas is probably most relevant for graphs, but here is how it works; it also changes the display of thousands delimiters:

```
. set dp comma
. list in 1/3, clean
          usd        eur        jpy
  1.    1645,82    1362,40    192.308
  2.   22628,54   18731,74  2.644.058
  3.   12693,05   10507,22  1.483.135
```

You can also specify a format as, e.g., %9,0g to display decimal commas, but it does not always work as expected. Remember that, no matter how you specify formats, in commands Stata understands only decimal periods.

The general rule is that format affects the display of single values, as in list, whereas output from analyses is displayed regardless of the format. There are, however, exceptions, and a fixed (f) format does influence the output from tabulate with the summarize() option, oneway with the tabulate option, and ci. In some other commands, such as tabstat (section 10.4), a format() option lets you determine the output format.

5.3 Missing values

> Find exercises about how to work with missing values in section 20.4.

Missing values are omitted from calculations and analyses. There are two types of missing values:

- *System missing values* are shown as a . (period). Such a value is created in input when a numeric field is empty; by invalid calculations, e.g., division by 0; and by calculations involving a missing value.

- *User-defined missing values* are .a, .b, .c, ..., .z. It is a good idea to use a general principle consistently, e.g.,

	Question not asked (complications to an operation not performed)
.a	Question asked, no response
.b	Response: Do not know

See [U] **12.2.1 Missing values** and [D] **missing values**. Coding missing information as missing is important for continuous variables. Ask yourself, Would it make any sense to calculate the mean for this variable? If not, as is the case for categorical variables, consider how you want to use information about nonresponses and do-not-know responses in your analyses. A "Do not know" answer is often as interesting as a "Yes", and in such cases do-not-know responses should not be coded as missing.

If you enter data in Stata's Data Editor, you may also enter these missing value codes, but probably no other data entry program accepts .a in a numeric field. (See section 6.2 for more information about entering data.) When entering data, you might choose the codes -1 to -3 (provided, of course, that they could not be valid codes) and let Stata recode them:

```
. recode _all (-1=.)(-2=.a)(-3=.b)
```

mvdecode (see [D] **mvencode**) does essentially the same thing:

```
. mvdecode _all, mv(-1=. \ -2=.a \ -3=.b)
```

If you need to export data to another program that does not understand Stata's missing value codes, you could perform the reverse process:

```
. recode _all (.=-1)(.a=-2)(.b=-3)
```

However, mvencode is safer because it will refuse to recode to a value that already exists in the dataset:

```
. mvencode _all, mv(.=-1 \ .a=-2 \ .b=-3)
```

Precautions with missing values

You need not bother about the actual numerical values behind the missing values, but you need to know the logic to avoid mistakes. (See [U] **12.2.1 Missing values** for more information.) Missing values are high-end numbers; the ordering is

> all valid numbers $< . < .a < .b < \cdots < .z$

Calculations involving one or more missing values lead to a missing result, and missing values are omitted from analyses, but the situation is different for logical expressions. The expression age>65 is true for an observation with missing age. Stata's behavior is predictable once you make this clear to yourself, but a warning is warranted.

Warning: Missing values in logical expressions

The following command initially surprised me by listing all whose ages were greater than 65 *and* those with a missing age:

```
. list id age if age > 65
```

Technically, a missing value is larger than any valid number, which means that the expression age > 65 is true if age is missing. To exclude the missing values, type

```
. list id age if age > 65 & age < .
```

or

```
. list id age if age > 65 & ! missing(age)
```

To list the missing values only, including user-defined missing values, type

```
. list id age if age >= .
```

or

```
. list id age if missing(age)
```

5.4   Storage types and precision

Numeric variables can be integers (no decimals) and floating-point numbers (with decimals); see table 5.2. Integers come in three sizes: byte, int, and long. Floating-point numbers come in two sizes: float and double (double precision). Calculations are performed in double precision, but the default storage type of the result is float, as a compromise between precision and storage use. Read more in [U] **12.2.2 Numeric storage types**.

Table 5.2. Storage types of numeric variables

Variable type	Storage type	Bytes	Precision (digits)	Approx. range
Integer	byte	1	2	± 100
	int	2	4	$\pm 32{,}000$
	long	4	9	$\pm 2 \times 10^9$
Floating point	float	4	7	$\pm 10^{38}$
	double	8	16	$\pm 10^{307}$

With large numbers, you may have problems with precision, as demonstrated in the following example:

```
. clear
. set obs 1                              Generate an empty observation
obs was 0, now 1
. generate xfloat=999999^2               A float (4-byte) variable
. generate double xdouble=999999^2       A double (8-byte) variable
. generate long xlong=999999^2           A long (4-byte) integer
. format xfloat-xlong %12.0f             Define display format
. list, clean
         xfloat       xdouble    xlong
  1.   999998029824  999998000001       .
```

xdouble shows the correct result; it is defined to be double precision. xfloat has the default float storage type; it is correct up to the first seven digits only. xlong is a long integer with a maximum of nine digits, too few for the result, which becomes missing.

set obs 1 sets the number of observations in memory to 1. This is a necessary step to generate variables when there is no dataset in memory. For more information, see [D] **obs**.

You can see the storage types for the variables in a dataset with describe:

```
. describe
Contains data
  obs:             1
  vars:            3
  size:           20 (99.9% of memory free)

                storage  display    value
variable name   type     format     label      variable label

xfloat          float    %12.0f
xdouble         double   %12.0f
xlong           long     %12.0f

Sorted by:
    Note:  dataset has changed since last saved
```

The following gives another illustration:

```
. clear
. set obs 1                          Create an empty observation
obs was 0, now 1
. generate xf = 1/7                  xf is float; 1/7 is double
. generate double xd = 1/7           xd is double; 1/7 is double
. list if xf == 1/7, clean
    (nothing happened)               xf (float) is not equal to 1/7 (double)
. list if xd == 1/7, clean           xd (double) is equal to 1/7 (double)
        xf          xd
1.   .1428571    .14285714
```

Although we generated xf=1/7, the relational expression xf==1/7 was not true. xf is a float (4 bytes), while 1/7 during calculation is a double (8 bytes). Because of precision problems, xf and 1/7 were not equal. For the double-precision xd, the expression xd==1/7 was true. The expression xf==float(1/7) would be true, too.

The default float storage type uses 4 bytes per variable per observation, but variables often take small integer values only. They can be stored as a byte storage type. The command

```
. compress
```

finds the smallest possible storage type for each variable, and this can substantially reduce memory requirements without compromising precision; see section 5.7 about memory considerations.

5.5   Date and time variables

Date and time variables are numeric variables which can be displayed in a special format. The numeric value of a date variable is the number of days since 1 January 1960; the value of dates before that is negative. The numeric value of a date-and-time variable is the number of milliseconds since midnight on 1 January 1960. You may generate variables with other units such as weeks, months, and quarters; however, they are not described in this book. Read more in [U] **24 Dealing with dates and times**, [U] **12.5.3 Date and time formats**, and [D] **dates and times**, or use the online help by typing

```
. help date
```

Find exercises about how to work with date variables in section 20.5.

Date formats

Format specifications for dates start with %td. Specifying %td only is equivalent to specifying %tdDDmonCCYY, displaying a date as 19oct1993. To display this date as 19.10.1993, specify the format %tdDD.NN.CCYY (DD for day, NN for numeric month, CC for century, YY for two-digit year). To display it as 10/19/1993 the format is %tdNN/DD/CCYY.

```
. clear
. set obs 1
obs was 0, now 1
. generate d1=12345
. generate d2=d1
. generate d3=d1
. generate d4=d1
. format d2 %td
. format d3 %tdDD.NN.CCYY
. format d4 %tdNN/DD/CCYY
. list, clean
            d1        d2          d3          d4
   1.    12345   19oct1993   19.10.1993   10/19/1993
```

Prior to Stata 10, date format descriptors started with %d. Stata 10 still understands the old format descriptors, but that may not be the case with future Stata versions, unless you use version control; see section 4.9.

Generating date variables

The numeric value of a date can be calculated from three variables: day (bd), month (bm), and year (by). The mdy() function requires the sequence to be month, day, year:

```
. generate bdate = mdy(bm,bd,by)
. format bdate %td
```

You can translate a date written as a string variable (sbdate) to a date variable. The date() function "understands" many input formats: "17jan2001", "17/1/2001", "17.1.2001", "17 01 2001", and even "17012001". The sequence of arguments is defined by a mask; here "DMY" defines the sequence day, month, year.

```
. generate bdate = date(sbdate,"DMY")
. format bdate %td
```

In general, enter and display four-digit years to avoid ambiguity about the century. If you received data with two-digit years, you can make sure that the data are interpreted as lying between, e.g., 1911 and 2010:

```
. generate bdate = date(sbdate,"DMY",2010)
```

This means that the year must be 2010 or earlier, so 9 will be interpreted as 2009, 10 as 2010, and 11 as 1911.

Calculations with dates

The length of a time interval can be calculated as the difference in days between the last date (date2) and the first date (date1):

```
. generate days = date2 - date1
```

To express the length of a time interval in years:

```
. generate years = (date2 - date1)/365.25
```

This technique to express a time interval in years is fine for, e.g., survival analysis. For legal purposes, the method can be troublesome because of the effect of leap years. Legally, a person who was born 15 March 1989 became 18 years old on 15 March 2007. But, according to the above calculation technique, he was not quite 18 years old until the next day. It is outside the scope of this book to show how to handle this kind of problem.

You may extract day, month, and year from a date variable (bdate):

```
. generate bday = day(bdate)
. generate bmonth = month(bdate)
. generate byear = year(bdate)
```

Date-and-time variables

To include the time of day, use the %tc (c for clock) format rather than the %td format. A %tc value is the number of milliseconds since the start of 1 January 1960, but it can be displayed in a legible way, controlled by the %tc format. If you work with time intervals finer than hours, you must store your date-and-time variables as double to avoid precision problems. In the following example, datetime2 should be the same as datetime1, but it is actually 8 seconds off.

```
. clear
. set obs 1
obs was 0, now 1
. generate double datetime1 = 394839482000
. generate float datetime2 = datetime1
. format datetime? %tc
. list, clean

              datetime1            datetime2
   1.    05jul1972 21:38:02   05jul1972 21:38:10
```

A date-and-time variable can be entered in a more legible way than the large integer above:

```
. generate double datetime = tc(05jul1972 21:38)
```

You can generate a date-and-time variable from its components, in the sequence month (bm), day (bd), year (by), hours (bhour), minutes (bmin), and seconds (bsec). If the seconds are not recorded, you can include a constant.

```
. generate double bdatetime = mdyhms(bm, bd, by, bhour, bmin, 0)
. format bdatetime %tc
```

You can convert a string variable (sdatetime) containing date and time information with the clock() function. You need to define a mask to identify the sequence; here "DMYhm" defines the sequence day, month, year, hours, and minutes:

```
. generate double bdatetime = clock(sdatetime, "DMYhm")
. format bdatetime %tc
```

If you do not need the date but only the time of day, you can use a time variable, which has the internal value of milliseconds since midnight. Specify a format that omits the date component:

```
. generate double time = hms(21,38,0)
. format time %tcHH:MM
. list, clean

              time
  1.     21:38
```

Actually, if you display it with the general %tc format, you will see that the date is set to 1 January 1960, but because only the time of day is of interest, this is not a problem.

From two time variables or two date-and-time variables, you can calculate the length of a time interval much as you can with date variables. You might prefer to express the interval in hours rather than milliseconds:

```
. generate hours = (datetime2 - datetime1)/(60*60*1000)
```

You can extract hours, minutes, and seconds from a time variable or a date-and-time variable (datetime)

```
. generate hours = hh(datetime)
. generate minutes = mm(datetime)
. generate seconds = ss(datetime)
```

Other time units

Stata also handles weeks (%tw), months (%tm), quarters (%tq), and half-years (%th). In all cases, the numeric value is the number of units since the first week, month, quarter, or half-year of 1960. These units may be especially useful for time-series analysis; see the *Time-Series Reference Manual* ([TS]).

5.6   String variables

Throughout this text, I have demonstrated the use of numeric variables, but Stata also handles string (text) variables. It is almost always easier and more flexible to use numeric variables, but sometimes you might need string variables. Read more in [U] **12.4 Strings** and [U] **23 Dealing with strings**. Read about string functions in [D] **functions**.

String values must be enclosed in quotes, as in, for example,

```
. replace ph=45 if nation == "Danish"
```

Because of case sensitivity, "Danish", "danish", and "DANISH" are different string values.

A string can include any character and number; however, number strings are not interpreted by their numeric value, just as a sequence of characters. Strings are sorted in dictionary sequence; however, all uppercase letters come before lowercase, numbers come before letters, and spaces or blanks come before anything else. This principle also applies to relations: " " < "12" < "2" < "A" < "AA" < "Z" < "a".

Do not confuse string variables with value labels for numeric variables. When you list observations without the nolabel option, the listed labels look the same as a string variable, but they are not. Use describe to see the variable type. In the Data Editor, string variables are displayed in red, and value labels are in blue.

String formats

%10s displays a 10-character string, right-justified; %-10s displays it left-justified. For example,

```
. format patid %10s
```

Reading string variables into Stata

In the commands that read ASCII data (see section 6.3), the default data type is numeric, and string variables must be declared in the input command. str5 means a five-character text string:

```
. infix id 1-4 str5 icd10 5-9 using "a.txt"
```

Generating new string variables

The first time a string variable is defined, it can, but need not, be declared by its length (here str10):

```
. generate str10 nation = "Danish" if ph==45
```

This will work, too:

```
. generate nation = "Danish" if ph==45
```

Conversion between string and numeric variables

Numeric strings to numbers

If a 10-digit number is stored in idstr (type string), no calculations can be performed. You could convert it to the numeric variable idnum by typing

```
. generate double idnum = real(idstr)
. format idnum %010.0f
```

If the string variable contains decimal commas, the dpcomma option ensures that they are converted correctly to decimal numbers with periods:

```
. destring ss, generate(nn) dpcomma
```

idnum is a 10-digit number and must be declared double for sufficient precision (see section 5.4). The leading zero in the format descriptor tells Stata to display leading zeros, if any.

Another possibility is destring (see [D] **destring**), which automatically stores idnum as a double if needed:

```
. destring idstr, generate(idnum)
. format idnum %010.0f
```

Nonnumeric strings to numbers

If a string variable sex were coded as "M" and "F", you could convert it to a numeric variable, gender (with the original string codes as value labels), by typing

```
. encode sex, generate(gender)
```

encode will assign numeric codes in the string variable's alphabetic order. See [D] **encode**. You can, however, determine which strings get which codes by defining the value labels first:

```
. label define sexlbl 1 "M" 2 "F"
. encode sex, generate(gender) label(sexlbl)
```

Numbers to strings

You want to convert the numeric variable idnum to a string variable, idstr. If you want any leading zeros to be included in the string, specify the format "%010.0f":

```
. generate idstr = string(idnum, "%010.0f")
```

Another possibility is tostring (see [D] **destring**):

```
. tostring idnum, generate(idstr) format(%010.0f)
```

String manipulations

You can add (concatenate) strings with the + operator:

```
. clear
. set obs 1                          Generate empty observation
obs was 0
. generate svar3 = "abc"             Generate a 3-character string
. generate svar2 = "de"              Generate a 2-character string
. generate svar5 = svar3 + svar2     Add the strings
. list, clean
        svar3    svar2    svar5
   1.     abc       de    abcde
```

You can isolate part of a string variable with the `substr()` function. The arguments are source string, start position, and length. In the following, a3 will be characters 2–4 of `svar5`:

```
. generate a3 = substr(svar5,2,3)
. list, clean
        svar3    svar2    svar5    a3
   1.     abc       de    abcde    bcd
```

The `upper()` function converts lowercase characters to uppercase characters; the `lower()` function does the opposite. Imagine that ICD-10 codes had been entered inconsistently, with the same code sometimes as E10.1 and sometimes as e10.1. These are different strings, and you want them to be the same (E10.1):

```
. replace dx = upper(dx)
```

Handling complex strings, e.g., ICD-10 codes

In the International Classification of Diseases, 10th Revision (ICD-10), all codes are a combination of letters and numbers (e.g., E10.1 for insulin-demanding diabetes with ketoacidosis). This format is probably convenient for the person coding diagnoses (an important consideration), but for data management, it is inconvenient. I suggest splitting a five-character ICD-10 string variable (e.g., scode) into a one-character string variable (e.g., scode1) and a four-digit numeric variable (e.g., ncode4) by typing

```
. generate str1 scode1 = substr(scode,1,1)
. generate ncode4 = real(substr(scode,2,4))
. format ncode4 %4.1f
```

We obtained two variables: the string variable scode1 with 26 values (A–Z) and the numeric variable ncode4 (0.0–99.9). Now you can identify diabetes (E10.0–E14.9) by typing

```
. generate diab = 0
. replace diab = 1 if scode1 == "E" & ncode4 >= 10 & ncode4 < 15
```

If you received ASCII data, you could have obtained the same result by letting the `infix` command read the same data twice as different types:

```
. infix id 1-4 str5 scode 5-9 str1 scode1 5 ncode4 6-9 using
> "list1.txt"
```

You could also have identified diabetes by typing

```
. replace diab = 1 if scode >= "E10" & scode < "E15"
```

Here is another example: Say that you received raw information from a hospital discharge register, where all ICD-10 codes had a D prefix, code lengths varied, and the decimal point was not included:

```
. list in 1/3
```

	diag
1.	DI73
2.	DI739
3.	DI739A

To reformat the codes to a conventional format, you could use the `substr()` function. `substr(diag,5,.)` means from character 5 to the end, and `%-6s` left-justified the string:

```
. generate diag1 = substr(diag,2,3) + "." + substr(diag,5,.)
. format diag1 %-6s
. list in 1/3
```

	diag	diag1
1.	DI73	I73.
2.	DI739	I73.9
3.	DI739A	I73.9A

5.7   Memory considerations

In Stata/IC, a dataset can have a maximum of 2,047 variables; Stata/SE and Stata/MP can have 32,767. Stata keeps the entire dataset in memory, and the number of observations is limited by the memory allocated. The memory must be allocated before you load data into memory.

If the memory allocated is insufficient, you get the following message:

```
no room to add more observations
```

You may increase the current memory (e.g., to 25 MB) by typing

```
. clear
. set memory 25m [, permanently]
```

You can see the amount of used and free memory by typing

    `. memory`

If you allocate too much memory to Stata, you may make it slow down rather than improve its performance, so do not increase the memory allocated more than is needed. You can read more in [D] **memory** and [U] **6 Setting the size of memory**.

compress

See [D] **compress**. To reduce the physical size and memory requirements of your dataset, Stata can determine the smallest storage type needed for each variable (see section 5.4), and you can safely type

    `. compress`

and save the data again (`save, replace`). This step may reduce the memory needed by up to 80%.

Handling huge datasets

If you are handling a huge dataset, you may consider working on a subset of variables. Most often, you do not make analyses using all variables:

    `. use var1-var27 using hugeset.dta`

You may consider increasing your computer's RAM (not expensive). For instance, with 2 GB of RAM, you could `set memory 800m` for Stata, and this allocation would fit very large datasets, e.g., a million observations with 200 variables. Stata/SE can handle up to 32,767 variables, but memory restrictions otherwise do not differ from those of Stata/IC. Thirty-two–bit processors cannot handle more than 2 GB of RAM, and Windows XP has some further limitations; see the FAQ http://www.stata.com/support/faqs/win/winmemory.html. With the new 64-bit processors, the amount is virtually infinite. To benefit from this increase, you must also purchase a 64-bit Stata version; see http://www.stata.com/products/opsys.html.

You might want to `compress` a huge dataset, but you cannot load it because of its large size. Try to read one part of the data, compress and save, read the next part of the data, compress and save, etc., and finally combine (`append`) the partial datasets (see section 9.5). The following do-file shows what this series of steps might look like.

```
──────────────────────────── gen_aacomp.do ────────────────────────────
* gen_aacomp.do

cd C:\docs\proj1

use in 1/10000 using aa.dta, clear
compress
save aa1.dta

use in 10001/20000 using aa.dta, clear
compress
save aa2.dta

use in 20001/30000 using aa.dta, clear
compress

append using aa1.dta
append using aa2.dta
save aacomp.dta
```

If you encounter problems, carefully read [D] **memory**. Also read the FAQs on memory requirements for Windows (http://www.stata.com/support/faqs/win/); there are similar FAQs for other platforms.

6 Getting data in and out of Stata

6.1 Opening and saving Stata data

Precautions

When you open (use) a Stata dataset, you copy the contents of a disk file to the computer's memory (RAM). You can do any manipulation with the version in memory. It does not affect the contents of the disk file until you copy the version in memory back to the disk (save). It is like working with a word processor; you can write anything, but if you do not save the text before exiting, it has no permanent effect.

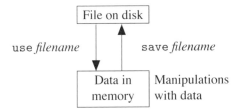

This is how most of us use a word processor. But have you ever, by mistake, overwritten good text with something else? I have. When it comes to your own data, collected at high expense, the cost of such a mistake may be high in terms of hours of work, or — worse — data loss or erroneous results. I strongly recommend the following principles:

- If you did not modify your data in memory, there is no point in saving them again.

- If you made modifications worth saving, save the revised data with a new filename to avoid overwriting the original data. You might have made mistakes, and overwriting existing data might destroy valuable information.

- Make modifications worth saving with a do-file, including the initial use command, the modifying commands, and the final save command. This do-file documents what you did, and if you made any errors, you can correct the do-file and run it again.

- To avoid mistakes, specify the full file path when using and saving files. This can be done in two ways

```
. cd C:\docs\proj1
. use example1.dta
. save example2.dta
```

or

```
. use C:\docs\proj1\example1.dta
. save C:\docs\proj1\example2.dta
```

Read more about such precautions in chapter 18. The principle can be illustrated like this

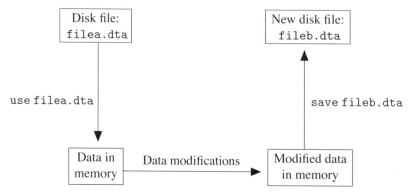

Defining the file path

Any survivors from the DOS era will recognize these commands, described in [D] **cd** and [D] **mkdir**. cd stands for change directory. Instead of specifying the full path in the use and save commands, you could do it with cd by typing

```
. cd C:\docs\proj1
. use example1.dta
```
(modifications to the data in memory)
```
. save example2.dta
```

cd defines the working directory, and its name is displayed in the lower-left corner of Stata's main window. You can also see it with the pwd command. cd .. (space between cd and ..) moves up one directory. mkdir (make directory) creates a new directory. A sequence of commands could return the following output:

. **pwd**	Display current directory
`C:\docs`	
. **cd proj2**	Change to the `proj2` subdirectory
`C:\docs\proj2`	
. **use example1.dta**	Use example1.dta in current directory
(commands modifying data)	
. **save example2.dta**	Save example2.dta in current directory
`file example2.dta saved`	
. **cd ..**	Move up one directory level
`C:\docs`	
. **mkdir proj3**	Create new subdirectory called `proj3`

If you use this method to define the file path, by all means include the `cd` command with the full path in every do-file; otherwise, the file location is undefined with the risk of major mistakes.

use

The use command is documented in [D] **use**.

Copy an existing Stata dataset from disk to memory by typing

```
. cd C:\docs\proj1
. use example1.dta
```

or, alternatively

```
. use C:\docs\proj1\example1.dta
```

If there are data in memory, use will be rejected unless you specify the clear option. You can also issue the clear command before the use command to delete the data in memory.

```
. use example1.dta, clear
```

or

```
. clear
. use example1.dta
```

Instead of typing the use command, you can click on the 🗋 button or select **Open...** from the **File** menu.

If you want to use only observations that meet a certain condition, type, for example,

```
. use example1.dta if sex==1
```

If you want only the first 100 observations, type

```
. use example1.dta in 1/100
```

If you want to work with a subset of variables, type, for example,

. `use age sex q1-q17 using example1.dta`

In this book, you will meet two special `use` commands:

. `sysuse auto.dta`   Use a dataset that is part of your Stata installation
. `webuse lbw.dta`   Use a dataset available over the Internet

save

The `save` command is documented in [D] **save**.

Save the data in memory to a disk file by typing

. `cd C:\docs\proj1`
. `save example2.dta`

or, alternatively

. `save C:\docs\proj1\example2.dta`

If you already have saved a file with this name, you will need to use the `replace` option. This measure is a safeguard against destroying your data on disk. Use the `replace` option only if you really want to overwrite data. Here is a typical situation: You are developing a do-file ending with a `save` command, and you need to modify your first attempts, so you need to use the `replace` option:

. `save example2.dta, replace`

`save` does not allow restrictions to a subset of observations or variables. Use the `keep` command (see section 9.2) if that is what you want by typing, for example,

. `keep age sex q1-q17`
. `save example2.dta, replace`

Instead of typing the `save` command, you can click on the ⊞ button or select Save As... from the File menu.

The file format created by Stata 10 is different from the Stata 9 format, and Stata 9 does not read a Stata 10 dataset. If you use Stata 10 and want to make a dataset available to a Stata 9 user, use the `saveold` command rather than the `save` command.

6.2   Entering data

In [U] **21 Inputting data** and [D] **infile**, you will find an overview of the different ways to enter data.

The input command

For small datasets, you can define the variables with the `input` command and enter the values. Finish the input with end. It can be done interactively from the command line or in a do-file. See [D] **input**, and see more examples in section 11.8 (*Graph examples*).

```
. clear
. input case expose pop
  0 0 100
  0 1 30
  1 0 23
  1 1 21
  end
```

Using Stata's Data Editor to enter data

You can use Stata's Data Editor to enter data in a spreadsheet format. A tutorial in the *Getting Started* manual describes one way to define the variables before entering data. I find it much easier to define the variables in a do-file, as shown in gen_aa0.do. Here we define id as a `string` variable, and type, sold, and price as numeric variables. This creates a template—a dataset with variables defined, but with no observations. You might also want to define variable labels and value labels (see chapter 7) at this stage.

```
─────────────────────── gen_aa0.do ───────────────────────
* gen_aa0.do
* Preparing to enter data in the Data Editor

cd "C:\docs\project aa"

clear
generate id=""
generate type=.
generate sold=.
generate price=.

save aa0.dta
```

Now you can use the Data Editor to enter data in the file. Use the *Tab* key to shift horizontally to the next variable. When you have entered the last variable in the first observation, use the *Enter* key to shift vertically to the next observation, and use the *Home* key to go left to the first variable. For the following observations, just use the *Tab* key; now the Data Editor knows the number of variables.

When you have finished a data-entry session, save the dataset with a new name, keeping the empty template unchanged; you may want to reuse it. It may be practical to save a separate file for each data-entry session and later append these files (see section 9.5).

For entering major amounts of data, the spreadsheet format is not optimal, and you should use a specialized program for data entry; see below.

Using a data-entry program

If you are going to enter many data, you will benefit from a specialized program for data entry. A good program for entering data should

- Enable you to set up a screen resembling, for example, a questionnaire page. This makes data entry easier and reduces the risk of errors (entering the right information in the wrong place).
- Check the validity of the data entered (checking that the data entered are within defined ranges).
- Enable you to enter data twice and compare the two files.
- Allow you to export data to the statistical program you use.

One such program is EpiData, which can be downloaded at no cost. It is easy to learn and easy to install. It can export data to Stata, SAS, SPSS, and spreadsheets. In section 18.5, I give some more advice about entering data.

At the web site for this book, you will find a short description of EpiData and instructions on obtaining it and using it to produce Stata datasets; see *Other supplementary materials provided by the author* at http://www.stata-press.com/books/ishr2.html.

6.3   Reading ASCII data

On decimal periods and commas

Stata cannot read or write ASCII data with decimal commas, regardless of the Windows settings. The Stata command `set dp comma` affects how values are displayed, not how they are written to or read from ASCII files.

If your computer displays decimal commas, I suggest that you change the Windows settings by selecting

> [Start] ▷ Control Panel ▷ Regional and Language Options

Here you can choose a country that uses decimal periods.

If you received an ASCII file with decimal commas from someone else, you could use a text editor to replace the commas with periods—but if the file has text strings including commas, then another problem is created. Another way around the problem, if the file is tab-delimited or semicolon-delimited, is to

1. Change the Windows settings to use decimal commas.
2. Import the text file to a spreadsheet program such as Excel.
3. Change the Windows settings to use decimal periods.
4. Export data as a tab-delimited text file; it now has decimal periods.

Reading tab- or comma-separated data

For more information about reading tab- or comma-separated data, see [D] **insheet**. In tab-separated data, the tab character, here displayed as <T>, separates the values. A tab-separated ASCII file is created, for example, if you save an Excel worksheet as a text (.txt) file. If row 1 has variable names, Stata will figure this out and use them, but the variable names must follow Stata's rules (no spaces or special characters).

In this example, called a.txt, the value of type in observation 2 is missing:

```
id<T>type<T>sold<T>price
1<T>2<T>47<T>51.23
2<T> <T>793<T>199.70
```

You can read a tab-separated ASCII file with variable names in row 1 by typing the command

```
. insheet using a.txt, tab
```

In comma-separated data, commas separate the values:

```
1,2,47,51.23
2, ,793,199.70
```

If you have a comma-separated file without variable names in row 1, you would use the command

```
. insheet id type sold price using a.txt, comma
```

and with any other separator (here a semicolon), you would use

```
. insheet id type sold price using a.txt, delimit(";")
```

insheet assumes that all data belonging to one observation are in one line.

Reading free-format data

See [D] **infile (free format)** for details on reading free-format data. In free-format data, commas or blank spaces separate the values:

```
1 2 47 51.23
2 . 793 199.70
```

The command for reading such data is

```
. infile id type sold price using a.txt
```

infile does not assume that data belonging to one observation are in one line. infile considers the following data to be the same as the data above:

```
1 2 47 51.23 2 . 793 199.70
```

Reading fixed-format data

For detailed information about reading fixed-format data, see [D] **infix (fixed format)**. In fixed-format data, the information on each variable is determined by the position in the line; these positions are defined in the infix command. The blank type in observation 2 will be read as missing.

```
12 47 51.23
2 793199.70
```

The command for reading these data is

```
. infix id 1 type 2 sold 3-5 price 6-11 using a.txt
```

Fixed-format data can also be read by infile. To do this, you must create a dictionary file, specifying variable names and positions, etc. See [D] **infile (fixed format)**.

6.4   Exchanging data with other programs

> Take care: Translation between programs may go wrong, so you should carefully compare the output from Stata's summarize and, e.g., SPSS's DESCRIPTIVES and compare the number of valid values for each variable and the minimum and maximum values. Be especially careful with missing values and date variables.

Translation programs

If you use more than one statistical program, or if you are switching from another program to Stata, you will need a program to translate your data. One such translation program is Stat/Transfer (available from Circle Systems). Variable names, variables, and value labels are transferred as part of the data. Stat/Transfer 9 translates Stata 10 files, but Stat/Transfer 8 does not. To create a Stata dataset for conversion by Stat/Transfer 7 or 8, type

```
. saveold filename.dta
```

Transferring data to Excel and other spreadsheets

Stata can save a dataset in XML format, which can be read by Excel (see [D] **xmlsave**):

```
. sysuse auto.dta
(1978 Automobile Data)
. xmlsave auto.xml, doctype(excel)
```

Before Stata 9, a more traditional method was needed (and it still works): create a tab-separated file with variable names in the first row to be read by a spreadsheet (see [D] **outsheet**):

> . outsheet [*varlist*] using *filename*.txt, nolabel

In Excel, open the file as a text file, and follow the instructions. Variable names, but not labels, are transferred. You can create a similar file without variable names in the first row by typing

> . outsheet [*varlist*] using *filename*.txt, nolabel nonames

If you want to write the data to a comma-separated ASCII file, use the command (see [D] **outfile**)

> . outfile [*varlist*] using *filename*.txt, nolabel comma

Make sure you set your Windows international settings to use decimal periods; see section 6.3.

Rather than looking up the commands, you might prefer to use the menu system. Start by selecting

> File ▷ Export

Reading spreadsheet data

Stata can read a dataset in XML format, which could be created by Excel (see [D] **xmlsave**). The `firstrow` option tells Stata to interpret the first row in the spreadsheet as variable names:

> . xmluse auto.xml, doctype(excel) sheet("Sheet1") firstrow

For this to work, the Excel worksheet must have a simple rectangular structure with variable names in the first row. Also, the variable names must fulfill Stata's requirements: they must be unique and not include spaces or special characters.

Prior to Stata 9, a more traditional method was needed (and it still works); see [D] **insheet**. Many packages can create Excel data and most can create text files like those created by Stata's `outsheet` command. In Excel, you save a tab-separated text file (e.g., a.txt); Stata reads it when you type

> . insheet using a.txt, tab

Rather than looking up the commands, you might prefer to use the menu system. Select

> File ▷ Import

Copying and pasting between a spreadsheet and Stata's Data Editor

Copying and pasting between a spreadsheet and Stata's Data Editor works almost by intuition. But beware that the risk of errors is rather high, and you may encounter problems with variable types. For example, a variable that should be numeric is converted to a string variable. Again, Windows should be set to display decimal periods; otherwise, it will not work right.

There is an FAQ about this topic by N. J. Cox: *How do I get information from Excel into Stata?*. You can find it at http://www.stata.com/support/faqs/data/newexcel.html.

ODBC: Open DataBase Connectivity

odbc allows Stata to load data from ODBC sources, such as certain databases. You can read more in [D] **odbc**.

Translation between SAS and Stata using FDA file formats

fdasave and fdause convert datasets to and from the U.S. Food and Drug Administration's (FDA) SAS format for new drug and device applications. The primary intent of these commands is to assist people in making submissions to the FDA, but the commands are general enough to use in transferring data between SAS and Stata. Read more in [D] **fdasave**.

7 Documentation commands

Documentation commands let you add explanatory text to your data. A dataset label gives you descriptive information when you open the dataset. Variable labels and value labels add explanatory text to output from analyses.

You do not need documentation commands to analyze data, but using them will help make your output legible and reduce the risk of errors when interpreting the output.

7.1 Labels

You can read more about labels in [D] **label**.

Dataset label

You can give a short description of your data to be displayed every time you open (use) the dataset by typing, for example,

```
. label data "Fertility data Denmark 1997-99. ver 2.5, 19sep2002"
```

Include the creation date to be sure of which version you are analyzing.

Variable labels

You can attach explanatory text to a variable name similarly, for example,

```
. label variable q6 "Ever itchy skin rash?"
```

Use informative labels, but make them short. Long variable labels are often abbreviated in output.

Value labels

You can attach explanatory text to each code for a categorical variable. This is a two-step procedure. First, define the label (using double quotes around text with embedded spaces):

    . label define sexlbl 1 male 2 female 9 "sex unknown"

Next associate the label sexlbl with the variable sex:

    . label values sex sexlbl

Use informative labels, but make them short. Value labels are often abbreviated to 12 characters in output.

Most often, you will use the same name for a variable and its label:

    . label define sex 1 male 2 female
    . label values sex sex

But one label can be used for several variables:

    . label define yesno 1 yes 2 no
    . label values q1-q15 yesno

If you want to modify a label definition or add new labels, use the modify option:

    . label define sexlbl 9 "unknown sex", modify

In output, Stata displays either the value labels or the codes (when you specify the nolabel option). However, you often need to see them both to avoid mistakes. You can do so by including the codes in the labels by using the numlabel command; see [D] **labelbook**.

    . numlabel [lblname-list], add

Labels in multiple languages

A dataset can have more than one set of labels, e.g., an English set and a Spanish set, or you could have one set with long labels and another set with short labels. See [D] **label language** or type

    . help label language

See label definitions

codebook with the compact option displays the variable labels and other summary information about the variables. This command is most useful for obtaining an overview of a dataset:

```
. sysuse auto.dta, clear
(1978 Automobile Data)

. codebook, compact
Variable       Obs Unique      Mean    Min    Max  Label

make            74     74         .      .      .  Make and Model
price           74     74  6165.257   3291  15906  Price
mpg             74     21   21.2973     12     41  Mileage (mpg)
rep78           69      5  3.405797      1      5  Repair Record 1978
headroom        74      8  2.993243    1.5      5  Headroom (in.)
trunk           74     18  13.75676      5     23  Trunk space (cu. ft.)
weight          74     64  3019.459   1760   4840  Weight (lbs.)
length          74     47  187.9324    142    233  Length (in.)
turn            74     18  39.64865     31     51  Turn Circle (ft.)
displacement    74     31  197.2973     79    425  Displacement (cu. in.)
gear_ratio      74     36  3.014865   2.19   3.89  Gear Ratio
foreign         74      2  .2972973      0      1  Car type
```

Typing describe gives you more information on formats and labels:

```
. describe
Contains data from C:\Stata\ado\base\a\auto.dta
  obs:           74                           1978 Automobile Data
  vars:          12                           13 Apr 2007 17:45
  size:       3,478 (99.9% of memory free)  (_dta has notes)

              storage  display    value
variable name   type   format     label      variable label

make            str18  %-18s                 Make and Model
price           int    %8.0gc                Price
mpg             int    %8.0g                 Mileage (mpg)
  (output omitted )
foreign         byte   %8.0g      origin     Car type

Sorted by:  foreign
```

One variable (foreign) also has value labels (origin), which you can list by typing

```
. label list
origin:
          0 Domestic
          1 Foreign
```

Typing labelbook gives you more details about the labels; see [D] **labelbook**.

Typing codebook (without the compact option) gives you a lot of information for each variable (see section 10.1).

Notes

You can add notes to your dataset (see [D] **notes**):

```
. notes: 19oct2000. Corrections made after proofreading
```

You can also add notes to single variables:

```
. notes age: 20oct2000. Ages > 120 and < 0 recoded to missing
```

The notes are stored in the dataset; you can display them by typing

```
. notes
```

Notes are cumulative; old notes are not discarded, but you can drop notes by using the notes drop command (see [D] **notes**).

7.2 Working with labels: An example

In the auto.dta dataset, foreign is a strange variable name; I want to change it to origin. The variable label is Car type; I think Country of origin is a better choice. And living outside the United States, I want the value labels Domestic and Foreign replaced by U.S. and Other.

For this example, I begin by renaming the variable and removing the current labels:

```
. sysuse auto.dta
(1978 Automobile Data)
. rename foreign origin          See section 9.3
. label variable origin          Remove any variable label
. label drop origin              Drop value label origin
```

With no labels defined, a simple frequency table looks like this:

```
. tab1 origin
-> tabulation of origin
```

origin	Freq.	Percent	Cum.
0	52	70.27	70.27
1	22	29.73	100.00
Total	74	100.00	

This display is not very informative; you cannot see the meaning of origin or the meaning of the codes 0 and 1. Defining variable and value labels is helpful:

```
. label variable origin "Country of origin"
. label define origin 0 "U.S." 1 "Other"
. label values origin origin
```

```
. tab1 origin

-> tabulation of origin
```

Country of origin	Freq.	Percent	Cum.
U.S.	52	70.27	70.27
Other	22	29.73	100.00
Total	74	100.00	

Now the table displays explanatory text (Country of origin) and the meaning of the codes (U.S., Other) rather than the codes themselves (0, 1). This clarification makes the table easier to read and reduces the risk of mistakes. It would, however, be useful to see the codes and the value labels at the same time. You can do this by using the numlabel command:

```
. numlabel, add

. tab1 origin

-> tabulation of origin
```

Country of origin	Freq.	Percent	Cum.
0. U.S.	52	70.27	70.27
1. Other	22	29.73	100.00
Total	74	100.00	

Now you have all the information you need: you have defined the origin variable ("Country of origin") and its codes (0 is "U.S."; 1 is "Other"). Seeing the codes and the value labels together is useful, among other reasons because the if qualifier needs the code, not the value label.

```
. summarize if origin == "U.S."

type mismatch
r(109);
```

Stata did not understand your intent; the type mismatch message is due to a mismatch between the numeric variable origin and the string "U.S.". You must ask for the code, not the label:

```
. summarize if origin == 0
```

In the example shown, you should include the commands in a do-file. This file differs a bit from what you saw before, but it has the same effect.

(Continued on next page)

```
──────────────────────── gen_auto2.do ────────────────────────
* gen_auto2.do generates auto2.dta:  Revised labels

sysuse auto.dta
rename foreign origin                        // Change variable name
label variable origin "Country of origin"    // Define variable label
label define origin 0 "U.S." 1 "Other", modify  // Define value labels
label values origin origin                   // and apply to variable
numlabel origin, add                         // Add codes to value labels
compress                                     // A good place to do this

cd C:\docs\ishr2
save auto2.dta                               // Save revised dataset
```

The variable label and value label definitions are now included in auto2.dta. Adding or modifying labels is a modification of the dataset, so you should use a do-file that generates a dataset with a new name.

Chapter 18 will give you more advice and some more tools for documenting your data. As you have already seen, I favor using sensible variable names, informative labels, and do-files with names that tell what they do (gen_auto2.do generates auto2.dta).

8 Calculations

Calculation commands generate new variables or modify the values of existing variables. This chapter concerns numeric variables. String variables were explained in section 5.6.

Operators and functions for calculations are shown in section 8.2; you can also read more in [D] **generate** and [U] **13 Functions and expressions**.

> Section 20.3 contains exercises to help you get experience with some basic tools for calculation. These exercises also draw on commands explained in chapters 6 and 7.

8.1   generate and replace

Generate a new variable by typing, for example,

```
. generate bmi = weight/(height^2)
```

If the target variable (bmi) already exists in the dataset, generate will be rejected, and you must replace bmi by typing

```
. replace bmi = weight/(height^2)
```

The distinction between generate and replace is a safeguard to prevent you from unintentionally overwriting existing data. generate is one of the few commands I abbreviate (to gen); as a safeguard, replace cannot be abbreviated.

Using the if qualifier

You can use the if qualifier to restrict the calculations to a subset of data. To do calculations for males only, type, for example,

```
. generate mbmi = 1.1*bmi if sex==1   This is just an example
. replace npreg = . if sex==1         Number of pregnancies missing for males
                                          (question not asked)
```

Using the in qualifier

You can use the in qualifier to restrict the calculations to specific observations. This qualifier can be used, e.g., for corrections:

. `replace weight = 87 in 227`   Correction to observation 227

Using the by. . . : construct

You can use the by *varlist*: prefix, e.g., when numbering observations:

. `bysort sex: generate obsno = _n`   Consecutive numbering within each sex
                                        (example in section 8.5)

Calculations involving missing values

If a calculation involves a missing value, the result will be missing; for the calculations above, bmi will be missing if height or weight is missing.

Calculations involving logical expressions

If we want to use a BMI value to classify people as obese (BMI $\geq$ 30) or not obese (BMI $<$ 30), we can do so in several ways. One way is to use recode (see section 8.4):

. `recode bmi (30/max=1)(min/30=0), generate(obese)`

Another option is to do the following (be careful not to include missing BMIs as obese):

. `generate obese=0`
. `replace obese=1 if bmi>=30`
. `replace obese=. if bmi>=.`

You can use one command to obtain the same results as the previous three: the right-hand side of a calculation can be a logical expression that can evaluate to 0 (meaning false) or 1 (meaning true):

. `generate obese = bmi>=30`

The target variable (obese) takes the value 0 if bmi $<$ 30 and 1 if bmi $\geq$ 30. But take care: a missing value is a large number, and the expression will evaluate to true if bmi is missing. There are two ways to handle this problem; one is to let obese be false (i.e., 0) if bmi is missing:

. `generate obese = bmi>=30 & bmi<.`

Another option (and usually a more consistent option) is to let obese be missing if bmi is missing:

. `generate obese = bmi>=30 if bmi<.`

The three ways to handle a missing value in a logical expression are illustrated below:

```
. generate obese1 = bmi>=30
. generate obese2 = bmi>=30 & bmi<.
. generate obese3 = bmi>=30 if bmi<.
(1 missing value generated)
. list bmi obese*, clean
       bmi   obese1   obese2   obese3
  1.   29       0        0        0
  2.   31       1        1        1
  3.    .       1        0        .
```

A variable can be evaluated as a logical expression. In the `auto.dta` dataset, the variable `foreign` takes the value 0 for domestic cars and 1 for foreign cars, and you can type

```
. summarize if foreign          Foreign cars (foreign=1)
. summarize if !foreign         Domestic cars (foreign=0)
```

The value 0 evaluates to false, whereas any other value, including missing, evaluates to true, so be careful: the expression `foreign` will evaluate to true for observations with `foreign` missing.

For an instructive FAQ titled *What is true and false in Stata?*, by N. J. Cox, go to http://www.stata.com/support/faqs/data/trueorfalse.html.

Checking your results

When you have made any complex modifications, check to see if they worked as intended by typing, for example,

```
. list weight height bmi in 1/5
```

or

```
. browse weight height bmi in 1/5
```

Also type

```
. summarize bmi
```

and look at minimum and maximum values, applying your knowledge that BMI values less than 15 and more than 40 are unusual. Find some more techniques to check the correctness of your actions in section 8.5.

(*Continued on next page*)

8.2   Operators and functions in calculations
Arithmetic operators

There are five arithmetic operators; see [U] **13 Functions and expressions**. The order of operations is as shown in table 8.1. Power comes before multiplication and division, which come before addition and subtraction.

Table 8.1. Arithmetic operators

^	power
*	multiplication
/	division
+	addition
–	subtraction

Here are some examples:

```
. generate alcohol = beers + wines + spirits
. generate bmi = weight/(height^2)
```

The parentheses in the last command ensure that `height^2` is calculated before the division. Here, however, the parentheses are unnecessary because power takes precedence over division — but they do not cause any harm. For example,

```
. generate z = a+b/y
```

means the same as

```
. generate z = a+(b/y)
```

but is different from

```
. generate z = (a+b)/y
```

because the parentheses tell Stata to perform the addition before the division. When in doubt, use parentheses. Parentheses may also make the command more transparent to you. For transparency, you can also use spacing, but spacing does not change a Stata command, so

```
. generate z = a + b/y
```

means the same to Stata as

```
. generate z = a+b / y
```

Functions

Besides the operators shown, there are several functions available in Stata; see [D] **functions**. I show some examples with `generate` and some with `display` (see section 10.6), but they are the same functions. Here are some examples of functions:

Mathematical functions

. `generate y=abs(x)`	Absolute value: $|x|$
. `gen y=exp(x)`	Exponential, e^x
. `gen y=ln(x)`	Natural logarithm
. `gen y=log10(x)`	Base-10 logarithm
. `gen y=sqrt(x)`	Square root
. `gen y=int(x)`	Integer part of x; `int(5.8)` = 5; `int(-5.8)` = -5
. `gen y=floor(x)`	Rounding down; `floor(-5.8)` = -6
. `gen y=ceil(x)`	Rounding up; `ceil(5.8)` = 6
. `gen y=round(x)`	Nearest integer; `round(5.8)` = 6
. `gen y=round(x,0.25)`	`round(5.8,0.25)` = 5.75
. `gen y=mod(x1,x2)`	Modulus; the remainder after dividing x1 by x2
. `gen y=max(x1,...,xn)`	Maximum nonmissing value of arguments
. `gen y=min(x1,...,xn)`	Minimum value of arguments
. `gen y=sum(x)`	Cumulative sum from first to current observation
. `gen y=sign(x)`	Returns -1 if x $<$ 0; 0 if x $=$ 0, 1 if x $>$ 0, . if x is missing

Statistical functions

. `display chi2tail(`*df*`, `*chi2*`)`	`chi2tail(1, 3.84)` $=$ 0.05
. `display invchi2tail(`*df*`, `*Pr*`)`	`invchi2tail(1, 0.05)` $=$ 3.84
. `display normal(`*z*`)`	`normal(-1.96)` $=$ 0.025
. `display invnormal(`*Pr*`)`	`invnormal(0.025)` $=$ -1.96
. `display ttail(`*df*`, `*t*`)`	`ttail(20, 2.09)` $=$ 0.025
. `display invttail(`*df*`, `*Pr*`)`	`invttail(20, 0.025)` $=$ 2.09

_n, _N, and some other functions

. `gen y=_n`	_n is the observation number
. `gen y=_N`	_N is the number of observations in the dataset
. `gen y=cond(`*exp*`, `*a*`, `*b*`)`	Returns *a* if *exp* is true, *b* if *exp* is false
. `gen y=cond(x>z,1,-1)`	Returns 1 if x>z; otherwise, it returns -1
. `gen y=uniform()`	Returns a random number in the range $0-1$ (section 16.1)

There must be no space between the function name and the opening parenthesis enclosing the arguments:

This is wrong:	. `generate y=round (x)`
This is right:	. `generate y=round(x)`

Look in [D] **functions** or use `help functions` to find many other functions, such as trigonometric functions, for example,

```
. generate y = sin(x)
```

To see the online help for a function, include parentheses after the function name:

```
. help sin()
```

String functions are described in section 5.6, and date functions are covered in section 5.5.

8.3   Extended functions: egen

egen (extensions to generate) provides more functions; see [D] **egen**. egen has no alternative like replace, and if the target variable, e.g., meanage, already exists, you must choose another variable name or

```
. drop meanage
```

before resubmitting the egen command. Here are some examples:

Generating the same value for all observations

. egen meanage=mean(age)	Mean age across observations
. by sex: egen meanage=mean(age)	Mean age across observations, for each sex
. egen medage=median(age)	Median age across observations
. egen sumage=total(age)	Sum across all observations
. egen maxage=max(age)	Maximum nonmissing value of age across observations
. egen minage=min(age)	Minimum value of age across observations
. egen validage=count(age)	Number of nonmissing age across observations

The above functions generate variables that are constant across the dataset (or across each subset defined by by...:). Conceptually, using one of these functions is like spreading the information from a summarize across the dataset. Missing values are excluded from the calculations.

Generating individual values for each observation (each row)

. egen qmin=rowmin(q1-q17)	Minimum value of q1-q17 for this observation
. egen qmax=rowmax(q1-q17)	Maximum nonmissing value of q1-q17 for this observation
. egen qmean=rowmean(q1-q17)	Mean value of q1-q17 for this observation
. egen qsum=rowtotal(q1-q17)	Sum of q1-q17 for this observation
. egen qmiss=rowmiss(q1-q17)	Number of missing q1-q17 for this observation
. egen qvalid=rownonmiss(q1-q17)	Number of nonmissing q1-q17 for this observation

For the first four of the above functions, any missing values are excluded from the analysis. If there are at least five nonmissing values, and you want to calculate the mean, type

```
. egen qvalid = rownonmiss(q1-q17)
. egen qmean = rowmean(q1-q17) if qvalid > 4
```

Some of the above functions have cousins in the general Stata functions, but the above functions are slightly different. egen's rowmax() function takes a variable list but no other arguments. Stata's max() function can take constants and variables but not in variable-list format:

. egen vmax = rowmax(v1-v5)	rowmax() takes a variable list
. egen vmax = rowmax(v1 v2 v3 v4 v5)	egen forbids commas between arguments
. generate vmax = max(v1,v2,v3,v4,v5)	generate requires commas between arguments
. generate vmax = max(v1,v2,0)	max() also takes constant arguments

The group() function

The group() function lets you generate a new variable with all possible combinations of the categories of one or more variables. This may be useful when you want a stratified analysis with more than one variable defining the strata. If sex has two categories and race has three, racesex will get six categories:

```
. egen racesex = group(race sex), label
. cc low smoke, by(racesex)
```

See section 8.6 for an example of using group() to give numbers to patients who could have several hospital admissions.

The cut() function

The cut() function lets you create groups from a continuous variable. This is a convenient way to recode a continuous variable into intervals of equal width. The numeric list should include a large number (200). If it had not, ages 85 and older would have been recoded to missing. The code for an interval is its lower limit.

```
. egen agegr=cut(age), at(0 5(10)85 200)
```

age	agegr
$0 \le$ age < 5	0
$5 \le$ age < 15	5
$15 \le$ age < 25	15
$\cdots$	
$85 \le$ age < 200	85

With the label option, the value labels will be 0-, 5-, etc., and the codes themselves will be consecutive integers, starting at 0:

```
. egen agegr=cut(age), at(0 5(10)85 200) label
```

age	agegr	Value label
$0 \le$ age < 5	0	0-
$5 \le$ age < 15	1	5-
$15 \le$ age < 25	2	15-
$\ldots$		
$85 \le$ age < 200	9	85-

Another use of the cut() function is to create groups with approximately equal numbers of observations. Here there are five groups (quintiles):

```
. egen agegr=cut(age), group(5) label
```

I rarely use the group() option. I prefer to present groups with "natural" intervals, and the at() option (or recode; see section 8.4) lets me do that.

The egenmore functions

egen allows skilled and creative users to invent new, unofficial functions. egenmore is a library of such functions. You can install them by typing

```
. ssc install egenmore
```

8.4   Recoding variables

See [D] **recode** for details on recoding variables. recode is useful, for example, for modifying codes of a categorical variable, such as sex:

```
. recode sex (0=2)        sex was F:0, M:1; now it is M:1, F:2
```

But be aware, first, that the rule not to overwrite original data was violated, and second, that the value labels no longer match the codes. A good solution, which creates a new variable (gender) and defines value labels at once, is to type

```
. recode sex (1=1 "male") (0=2 "female"), generate(gender)
. numlabel gender, add
. label variable gender "Sex of respondent"
```

If the target variable (gender) already exists, you will get an error message, so you must choose another variable name or type

```
. drop gender
```

before resubmitting the recode command.

Another option, of course, is to define value labels the standard way:

```
. recode sex (0=2), generate(gender)
. label define gender  1 male  2 female
. label values gender gender
. numlabel gender, add
. label variable gender "Sex of respondent"
```

The important point is that you should define labels as soon as you create a new variable. It will never be easier than at that point. It will only be more difficult if you postpone it. If you do not create labels, the risk of making mistakes is high.

recode is also typically used to generate a new categorical variable (e.g., agegr) from a continuous variable (e.g., age). age is recorded in years, but with the precision of days, and we want to ensure that age 55.00 (at the birthday) goes to category 4:

```
. recode age (55/max=4)(35/55=3)(15/35=2)(min/15=1), generate(agegr)
```

The value 55 was specified in both the first and the second intervals, but the information was "taken" by the first. When recode intervals overlap, the first interval specified wins.

Again, labels for the new variable should be defined at once:

```
. recode age (55/max=4 "55+")(35/55=3 "35-54")(15/35=2 "15-34")
> (min/15=1 "-14"), generate(agegr)
. numlabel agegr, add
. label variable agegr "Age at admission, grouped"
```

> Important: The generate() option creates a new variable with the recoded informa-
> tion. With
>
> ```
> . recode age (55/max=4)(35/55=3)(15/35=2)(min/15=1)
> ```
>
> age would be recoded into itself, meaning that the original information in age would
> be destroyed. You should never destroy primary information but rather create a new
> variable with the recoded information. The generate() option enables you to do that.

A continuous variable could also be grouped using egen's cut() function; see section 8.3.

Here are some other recode examples:

`. recode x (2=0)`	Values not recoded left unchanged
`. recode x (2=0), generate(x2)`	Values not recoded transferred unchanged
`. recode x (2=0) if sex==1`	Observations not included (sex!=1) left unchanged
`. recode x (2=0) if sex==1, gen(x2)`	x2 set to missing if sex!=1

. `recode x (2=0) if sex==1, gen(x2) copyrest`	Values transferred unchanged if sex!=1
. `recode x (2=0)(1=1)(else=9) [, gen(x2)]`	Recode remaining values to 9
. `recode x (9=.)`	Recode 9 to system missing
. `recode x (.=9)`	Recode system missing to 9
. `recode x (missing=9)`	Recode any missing value to 9

8.5   Checking correctness of calculations

If you made modifications of any complexity, check at once to see whether it worked as intended. To check the recoding of, for example, sex into gender, type

> . `tab2 sex gender`

To check the recoding of age into agegr, type

> . `sort age`
> . `list age agegr  [, nolabel]`

or

> . `sort age`
> . `browse age agegr [, nolabel]`

The sorting makes it easy to concentrate on the critical ages $(15, 35, 55)$. You can make it even easier by making a separator line when agegr changes:

> . `list age agegr, sepby(agegr)`

You can also use `tabstat` (see section 10.4) to check a `recode` operation. Here it confirms that the groups were created as intended:

> . `tabstat age, by(agegr) stat(min max)`

```
Summary for variables: age
     by categories of: agegr (Age at admission, grouped)
```

agegr	min	max
1. -14	1.512984	12.14663
2. 15-34	15.81985	30.97835
3. 35-54	35.33162	53.82302
4. 55+	55.95621	65.34012
Total	1.512984	65.34012

The `assert` command lets you include the checking in a do-file; see [D] **assert**. If the assertion is true, nothing happens:

```
. assert agegr==1 if age<15
. assert agegr==2 if age>=15 & age<35
. assert agegr==3 if age>=35 & age<55
. assert agegr==4 if age>=55 & age<.
```

If the assertion is false, an error message is issued and further execution stops. (In the following example, I deliberately made an error in the `assert` command, just to illustrate.):

```
. assert agegr==3 if age>=35 & age<65
10 contradictions in 25 observations
assertion is false
r(9);
```

`assert` is especially useful when you are processing large amounts of data and wish to verify that all is going as expected. If, for instance, you want to check if there is information on the sex of each person in a dataset, you could

```
. assert sex<.
```

8.6   Numbering observations

The variable age in the third observation can be referred to as age[3]; for more information, see [U] **13.7 Explicit subscripting**. The principle is

age	Current observation
age[_n]	Current observation
age[1]	First observation
age[_N]	Last observation
age[_n-1]	Previous (lag) observation
age[_n+1]	Next (lead) observation
age[27]	Observation 27

The following is a valid command:

```
. generate x = age[27]
```

This command sets x to the same value in all observations. However, explicit subscripting cannot take place to the left of the equal-sign, so the following command is not valid:

```
. replace x[28] = 15
```

Instead, type

```
. replace x = 15 in 28
```

Here is an example: From a patient register, you have information about hospital admissions, one or more per person, identified by patid (a 10-digit personal ID) and admdate (admission date). You want to construct the following variables: obsno (observation number), patno (study ID), admno (admission number), and admtot (patient's total number of admissions).

The do-file gen_patnumbers.do uses subscripting. With the by: construct, _n and _N apply to each subgroup, and typing

```
. by patid: generate admtot = _N
```

generates the total number of admissions for each patient.

```
───────────────────────── gen_patnumbers.do ──────────────
* gen_patnumbers.do
cd C:\docs\ishr2
use admissions.dta

* Sort by patient and date of admission, and generate observation number
sort patid admdate
generate obsno = _n
label variable obsno "Observation number"

* Give each patient a number
egen patno = group(patid)
label variable patno "Patient number"

* Generate admission number and total admissions for each patient
by patid: generate admno = _n
label variable admno "Patient's admission number"
by patid: generate admtot = _N
label variable admtot "Patient's number of admissions"

save patnumbers.dta
```

The result is shown here:

```
. list patid admdate obsno patno admno admtot in 1/7, sepby(patno)
```

	patid	admdate	obsno	patno	admno	admtot
1.	0605401234	01may1970	1	1	1	3
2.	0605401234	16may1970	2	1	2	3
3.	0605401234	04mar1971	3	1	3	3
4.	1705401234	22feb1970	4	2	1	1
5.	2705401235	01jan1970	5	3	1	1
6.	2805402345	29jan1970	6	4	1	2
7.	2805402345	14jul1970	7	4	2	2

It worked as intended.

Now the number of patients is displayed as the maximum by typing

. `summarize patno`

To study first admissions, type

. *anycommand* `if admno==1`

To study final admissions, type

. *anycommand* `if admno==admtot`

And to see the distribution of the patients' number of admissions, type

. `tab1 admtot if admno==1`

9 Commands affecting data structure

Whereas chapter 8 was concerned with single variables, this chapter describes how to modify the structure of your data. Beginners should read sections 9.1–9.4 but might want to skip some of the more complex material later in this chapter.

9.1 Safeguarding your data

When you use commands that modify your data, they affect the data in memory, not the data on disk. If you want to save the modifications, save a file with a *new* name to avoid destroying information; see section 6.1.

If you modified your data, you must issue a new `use` command to retrieve the dataset as it was prior to the modification. However, `preserve` and `restore` (documented in [P] **preserve**) let you make temporary modifications and selections:

`. preserve`	Preserve a copy of the data currently in memory
`. keep if sex == 1`	The following analyses are for males only
(analyses)	
`. restore`	Reload the preserved dataset

9.2 Selecting observations and variables

You can read more about selecting observations and variables in [D] **drop**.

Selecting variables

You can remove variables from the data in memory by typing, for example,

```
. keep sex age-weight
```

or by typing

```
. drop sbp*
```

You can also select only part of the data when you open a dataset. For example,

```
. use sex age-weight using alpha.dta
```

Selecting observations

You can remove observations from the data in memory by typing, for example,

```
. keep if sex == 1
```

or

```
. drop if sex != 1
```

You can restrict the data in memory to the first 100 observations by typing

```
. keep in 1/100
```

You can select part of the data when you open a dataset by typing, for example,

```
. use alpha.dta if sex == 1
. use alpha.dta in 1/100
```

Random sampling

You can keep a 10% random sample of the observations by typing

```
. sample 10
```

You can keep a sample of exactly 57 observations by typing

```
. sample 57, count
```

Read more about sampling and random numbers in section 16.1.

9.3   Renaming and reordering variables

Renaming variables

You can change the name of a variable by typing, for example,

```
. rename gender sex
```

Here the variable name gender is changed to sex. Contents and labels are unchanged. You can read more in [D] **rename**.

Reordering variables

To change the sequence of variables in the dataset, use the order command. For example,

```
. order id age-weight
```

The new sequence of variables will be as defined, and any variables not mentioned will follow after the variables mentioned.

To order the variables alphabetically, use the command

```
. aorder
```

For more information, see [D] **order**.

9.4 Sorting data

To sort your data according to mpg (primary key) and weight (secondary key), type

```
. sort mpg weight
```

sort sorts only in ascending order.

gsort is more flexible, but it is slower. To sort by mpg (ascending) and weight (descending), type

```
. gsort mpg -weight
```

The by *varlist:* prefix and some commands like merge (see section 9.5) require sorted data. You might be confident that your data are in the correct sequence, yet you get the error message

```
not sorted
```

The problem is that Stata does not know that the sequence is correct. The solution is to sort the data. For more information about sorting, see [D] **sort** and [D] **gsort**.

9.5 Combining files

Appending files

Imagine that, instead of auto.dta, you have two datasets: domestic.dta with data on 52 domestic makes, and foreign.dta with data on 22 foreign makes. You want to combine them to combined.dta (74 observations). The two datasets have the same variables. It might help to visualize the process:

(Continued on next page)

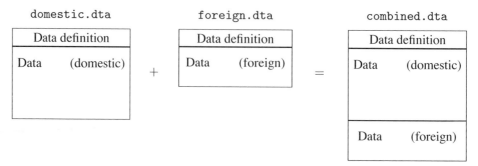

The two files have the same variables. It is only the data that differ. Combine the two files by using a do-file:

```
───────────────────── gen_combined.do ─────────────────────
* gen_combined.do
cd C:\docs\proj1
use domestic.dta
append using foreign.dta
save combined.dta
```

Here the dataset in memory before the append command was domestic.dta. This is called the master file or primary file. Labels from the secondary file (foreign.dta) will not replace labels in the master file, but if the master file has variables without labels, any labels from the secondary file will be copied—unless you specify the option nolabel. See [D] **append** for more about combining files.

Merging files

You might have information about individuals or other study objects from several sources. If the data from each source are in a separate file, you might want to combine them. The situation can be depicted like this:

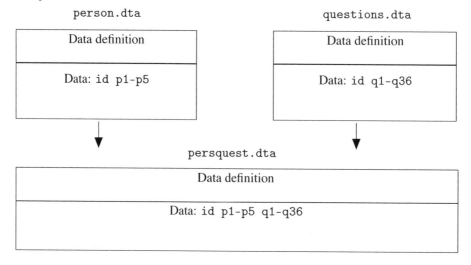

You have `person.dta` with the variables p1–p5 containing basic characteristics of the individuals, and `questions.dta` containing responses from a questionnaire in the variables q1–q36. In both datasets, the variable `id` uniquely identifies the individuals.

```
───────────────── gen_persquest.do ─────────────────
* gen_persquest.do

cd C:\docs\proj1
use person.dta
merge id using questions.dta, sort

save persquest.dta
```

The files must be sorted by the matching key (`id` in this example) before merging. You can accomplish this task by using the `sort` option. The matching key must have the same name in both datasets, but the other variable names should be different.

Stata creates the variable `_merge`, which takes the value 1 if its values come only from dataset 1 (`person.dta`), 2 if only dataset 2 (`questions.dta`) contributes, and 3 if both datasets contribute. If you expect no unmatched observations, check for mismatches with `assert` (see section 8.5):

```
. assert _merge==3
```

Get some more information by typing

```
. tab1 _merge
. list id _merge if _merge < 3
```

The `sort` option requires that the matching key be unique in both datasets, i.e., that there be no duplicate matching keys. If there are — and if that is not an error — do not use `merge`'s `sort` option, but use the `sort` command to sort both files by the matching key before merging.

In table 9.1, the matching key is not unique; there are duplicates. Numbers represent the matching key, and A and B represent the other variables in the input files. Missing information in the result file is shown by a period.

(Continued on next page)

Table 9.1. Matching key example

filea	fileb	fileab	_merge
1 A	1 B	1 A B	3
2 A		2 A .	1
	3 B	3 . B	2
4 A	4 B	4 A B	3
4 A		4 A B	3
5 A	5 B	5 A B	3
	5 B	5 A B	3

For id 4, there were two observations in the master file (filea) but only one in fileb, resulting in two observations with the information from fileb assigned to both of them. This method enables you to distribute information about patients to each of their admissions — if that is what you desire. But what if the duplicate id 4 was an error? To check for duplicate keys before merging, sort and compare with the previous observation:

```
. sort id
. list id if id==id[_n-1]
```

Another way to check for and list observations with duplicate IDs is to type

```
. duplicates report id
. duplicates list id
```

merge is a lot more flexible than described here. Among other things, you can use the using file to update the information in the master file; see [D] **merge**.

9.6   Reshaping data

contract, expand

contract *varlist* creates a dataset with an observation for each combination of values in *varlist*; the variable _freq indicates the frequency of each combination (see [D] **contract**). metricauto.dta includes the categorical variables foreign and mweightgr. Create a contracted dataset by typing

```
. cd C:\docs\ishr2
c:\docs\ishr2
. use metricauto.dta
(1978 Automobile Data)
. contract mweightgr foreign
```

The contracted dataset has 7 observations, one for each combination of mweightgr and foreign. The variable _freq is the number of observations for that combination:

```
. list, nolabel abbrev(10)
```

	foreign	mweightgr	_freq
1.	0	1	5
2.	1	1	12
3.	0	2	18
4.	1	2	9
5.	0	3	27
6.	1	3	1
7.	0	4	2

This is a tabular form of the data; you must use frequency weighting when analyzing such data:

```
. tab2 mweightgr foreign [fweight=_freq]
```

-> tabulation of mweightgr by foreign

Weight (kg) grouped	Car type 0. Domest	1. Foreig	Total
1. -999 kg	5	12	17
2. 1000-1499 kg	18	9	27
3. 1500-1999 kg	27	1	28
4. 2000 kg+	2	0	2
Total	52	22	74

With expand (see [D] **expand**), you can create the opposite effect; typing

```
. expand _freq
```

creates a dataset with 74 observations that can be analyzed without weighting.

Look at the example from section 4.5 about weighting observations. You have access to tabular information of the type in table 9.2.

Table 9.2. Tabular information about weighting observations

	Cases	Controls
Exposed	21	30
Unexposed	23	100
Total	44	130

You can create the corresponding contracted dataset by using the input command (see section 6.2):

```
. input expos case pop
  1 1 21
  1 0 30
  0 1 23
  0 0 100
  end
```

You can analyze by typing

```
. tab2 expos case [fweight=pop], chi2
```

See section 10.3 for more information about `tab2`.

You can obtain the same result by expanding the 4 observations to 174 observations:

```
. expand pop
. tab2 expos case, chi2
```

collapse

The `collapse` command (see [D] **collapse**) is similar to `contract`: you can use it to create an aggregated dataset, not with the characteristics of each individual but of groups of individuals. Imagine, for example, that you have data on the members of various trade unions. You now want to create a file characterizing each union by the proportion of males, by mean age, and by median income among members. `sex` is coded 0 for females, 1 for males.

```
. collapse (mean) meanage=age pmale=sex (median) medinc=income,
> by(union)
```

The aggregated dataset has one observation for each union, with the mean age, the proportion of males (the mean of a 0/1-coded variable is the proportion of 1s), and the median income.

A collapsed file like this one can again be merged with the original data to compare members with general characteristics of their union. The same comparison could be achieved by using the egen functions described in section 8.3:

```
. sort union
. by union: egen pmale = mean(sex)
. by union: egen meanage = mean(age)
. by union: egen medinc = median(income)
```

reshape

With repeated measurements and paired observations (not to mention dentistry, where a person may have 32 teeth), some analyses require a "wide" and some a "long" data structure. In `anklebp1.dta` (to be used again in chapter 15), the data structure is wide. One observation includes two blood-pressure measurements at each site:

```
. use anklebp1.dta
(Ankle blood pressure data)

. list in 1/3
```

	id	adp1	adp2	atp1	atp2
1.	1	105	110	105	105
2.	2	110	110	110	110
3.	4	140	130	150	160

For reasons explained in section 15.1, we need a long structure with one observation for each measurement:

```
. reshape long adp atp, i(id) j(meas)
(note: j = 1 2)
Data                                    wide   ->   long
```

	wide	->	long
Number of obs.	107	->	214
Number of variables	5	->	4
j variable (2 values)		->	meas
xij variables:			
	adp1 adp2	->	adp
	atp1 atp2	->	atp

The dataset now has the desired long structure with one observation per measurement:

```
. list in 1/6, sepby(id)
```

	id	meas	adp	atp
1.	1	1	105	105
2.	1	2	110	105
3.	2	1	110	110
4.	2	2	110	110
5.	4	1	140	150
6.	4	2	130	160

We could do the opposite by typing

```
. reshape wide adp atp, i(id) j(meas)
```

For more information, see [D] **reshape**. Also see a discussion of long and wide data structures in section 11.2 and an example of reshaping data in section 15.1.

separate

You can split a variable into two or more separate variables dependent upon the value of another categorical variable:

```
. sysuse auto.dta
(1978 Automobile Data)
. separate mpg, by(foreign)
```

variable name	storage type	display format	value label	variable label
mpg0	byte	%8.0g		mpg, foreign == Domestic
mpg1	byte	%8.0g		mpg, foreign == Foreign

```
. list foreign mpg*, nolabel sepby(foreign)
```

	foreign	mpg	mpg0	mpg1
1.	0	22	22	.
2.	0	17	17	.
3.	0	22	22	.

(Output omitted)

	foreign	mpg	mpg0	mpg1
53.	1	17	.	17
54.	1	23	.	23
55.	1	25	.	25

(Output omitted)

This may be practical for some types of graphs. Let's say we want to plot the relation between mileage and weight for foreign and domestic cars. The core command is

```
. twoway (scatter mpg weight if foreign==0)
> (scatter mpg weight if foreign==1)
```

With the two variables generated by separate, the graph command can be made simpler:

```
. twoway (scatter mpg0 mpg1 weight)
```

xpose

You can transpose observations and variables, changing observations to variables and variables to observations. This ability may be useful for restructuring data such as for use in a graph.

```
. xpose, clear
```

clear is mandatory to remind you that this command destroys your original data in memory. Read more in [D] **xpose**.

10 Description and simple analysis

In this chapter, I show the most important commands for description and simple analysis of data.

In section 20.6, you will find a number of exercises to get more experience with the commands explained in this chapter.

10.1 Overview of a dataset

The lbw dataset

For most analyses in this chapter, we will use the dataset lbw.dta from Hosmer and Lemeshow (2000) about predictors of low birthweight. The study was designed with an excess of children with low birthweight, but we will ignore that in this chapter. The dataset is used for several examples in the Stata reference manuals. You can obtain such datasets from the Internet by typing, for example,

```
. webuse lbw.dta
```

In this dataset, a common convention was used for yes–no variables: "No" is coded as 0 and "Yes" as 1. No value labels were defined for this rather obvious coding. I chose, however, to add value labels to these variables and save the dataset in C:\docs\ishr2 as lbw1.dta. Generally, you should make such modifications to the dataset using a do-file:

```
―――――――――――― gen_lbw1.do ――――――――――――
* gen_lbw1.do adds labels to lbw.dta and saves lbw1.dta

webuse lbw.dta

* Add value label yesno to the appropriate variables
label define yesno  0 No  1 Yes
label values low yesno
label values smoke yesno
label values ht yesno
label values ui yesno
numlabel _all, add                    // include code in value labels

* compress and save
compress
cd C:\docs\ishr2
save lbw1.dta
```

describe

describe (see [D] **describe**) gives you information about a dataset: the number of observations and variables, the file size in bytes, variable names, storage types (see section 5.4), display formats (see section 5.2), variable and value labels (see section 7.1), and the sorting status of the dataset. This dataset was not sorted:

```
. cd C:\docs\ishr2
c:\docs\ishr2

. use lbw1.dta
(Hosmer & Lemeshow data)

. describe

Contains data from lbw1.dta
  obs:           189                          Hosmer & Lemeshow data
  vars:           11                          2 Apr 2005 21:10
  size:         3,402 (99.9% of memory free)

              storage   display    value
variable name   type    format     label      variable label

id              int     %8.0g                 identification code
low             byte    %8.0g      yesno      birthweight<2500g
age             byte    %8.0g                 age of mother
lwt             int     %8.0g                 weight at last menstrual period
race            byte    %8.0g      race       race
smoke           byte    %8.0g      yesno      smoked during pregnancy
ptl             byte    %8.0g                 premature labor history (count)
ht              byte    %8.0g      yesno      has history of hypertension
ui              byte    %8.0g      yesno      presence, uterine irritability
ftv             byte    %8.0g                 number of visits to physician
                                                  during 1st trimester
bwt             int     %8.0g                 birthweight (grams)

Sorted by:
```

Use label list to see the value labels (the double numbers are due to numlabel, which added the code to the value label):

```
. label list
race:
           1 1. white
           2 2. black
           3 3. other
yesno:
           0 0. No
           1 1. Yes
```

codebook

codebook (see [D] **codebook**) gives you more detailed information about each variable. If you do not specify a variable list, Stata displays information for all variables, and the output may be a bit overwhelming. Here we ask for a single variable:

```
. codebook bwt
```

bwt					birthweight (grams)
type:	numeric (int)				
range:	[709,4990]			units:	1
unique values:	133			missing .:	0/189
mean:	2944.29				
std. dev:	729.016				

percentiles:	10%	25%	50%	75%	90%
	1970	2414	2977	3475	3884

The compact option is useful for obtaining an overview of the dataset. For each variable, this command displays the number of nonmissing observations, the number of unique values, and the minimum and maximum values:

```
. codebook, compact
```

Variable	Obs	Unique	Mean	Min	Max	Label
id	189	189	121.0794	4	226	identification code
low	189	2	.3121693	0	1	birthweight<2500g
age	189	24	23.2381	14	45	age of mother
lwt	189	76	129.8201	80	250	weight at last menstrual period
race	189	3	1.846561	1	3	race
smoke	189	2	.3915344	0	1	smoked during pregnancy
ptl	189	4	.1957672	0	3	premature labor history (count)
ht	189	2	.0634921	0	1	has history of hypertension
ui	189	2	.1481481	0	1	presence, uterine irritability
ftv	189	6	.7936508	0	6	number of visits to physician du...
bwt	189	133	2944.286	709	4990	birthweight (grams)

(Continued on next page)

summarize

summarize is another command that is useful for an initial overview of the data; see [R] **summarize**.

```
. summarize
    Variable |       Obs        Mean    Std. Dev.       Min        Max
-------------+--------------------------------------------------------
          id |       189    121.0794    63.30363          4        226
         low |       189    .3121693    .4646093          0          1
         age |       189     23.2381    5.298678         14         45
         lwt |       189    129.8201    30.57515         80        250
        race |       189    1.846561    .9183422          1          3
-------------+--------------------------------------------------------
       smoke |       189    .3915344    .4893898          0          1
         ptl |       189    .1957672    .4933419          0          3
          ht |       189    .0634921    .2444936          0          1
          ui |       189    .1481481    .3561903          0          1
         ftv |       189    .7936508    1.059286          0          6
-------------+--------------------------------------------------------
         bwt |       189    2944.286     729.016        709       4990
```

Most often, I prefer codebook, compact to summarize because it also displays the variable labels.

10.2   Listing observations

list

Listing observations is useful to help you examine data, check the results of calculations, and locate errors. Read more in [D] **list**. The following lists all variables in all observations:

```
. use lbw1.dta
(Hosmer & Lemeshow data)
. list

     +-----------------------------------------------------------------------------+
     | id    low   age   lwt      race   smoke   ptl      ht        ui   ftv   bwt |
  1. | 85   0. No   19   182   2. black   0. No     0   0. No   1. Yes     0  2523 |
  2. | 86   0. No   33   155   3. other   0. No     0   0. No   0. No      3  2551 |
  3. | 87   0. No   20   105   1. white   1. Yes    0   0. No   0. No      1  2557 |
  4. | 88   0. No   21   108   1. white   1. Yes    0   0. No   1. Yes     2  2594 |
  5. | 89   0. No   18   107   1. white   1. Yes    0   0. No   1. Yes     0  2600 |
     |-----------------------------------------------------------------------------|
  6. | 91   0. No   21   124   3. other   0. No     0   0. No   0. No      0  2622 |
     +-----------------------------------------------------------------------------+
                  (output omitted )
```

Often, listing the value labels creates more noise than clarity. To list the codes rather than the labels, use the nolabel option. Here we restrict to the variables id-smoke and to the first 5 observations:

```
. list id-smoke in 1/5, nolabel
```

	id	low	age	lwt	race	smoke
1.	85	0	19	182	2	0
2.	86	0	33	155	3	0
3.	87	0	20	105	1	1
4.	88	0	21	108	1	1
5.	89	0	18	107	1	1

You can get rid of the lines by using the clean option and drop observation numbers by using the noobs option:

```
. list id-smoke in 1/5, nolabel clean noobs
    id   low   age   lwt   race   smoke
    85    0    19    182    2      0
    86    0    33    155    3      0
    87    0    20    105    1      1
    88    0    21    108    1      1
    89    0    18    107    1      1
```

By default, list draws a separator line for each 5 observations. You can change this setting by using the separator() option. For example, separator(0) drops separator lines, whereas separator(10) draws a line for each 10 observations. The sepby(*varlist*) option draws a separator line each time the values in *varlist* change. The mean, sum, and N options (capital N) display a bottom line with the requested statistic. N displays the number of nonmissing values for each variable. If you supply a varlist, as in mean(bwt), the statistic will apply only to these variables.

```
. sort race smoke
. list race smoke bwt if bwt<1800, sepby(race) N mean(bwt)
```

	race	smoke	bwt
5.	1. white	0. No	1021
89.	1. white	1. Yes	1790
109.	2. black	0. No	1701
117.	2. black	1. Yes	1135
133.	3. other	0. No	1588
142.	3. other	0. No	1588
150.	3. other	0. No	1474
153.	3. other	0. No	1330
177.	3. other	0. No	1729
185.	3. other	1. Yes	709
Mean			1406.5
N	10	10	10

When you need to list more variables than can fit on a line, the `list` output becomes less useful:

```
. sysuse auto.dta
(1978 Automobile Data)
. list in 1/2, nolabel
```

1.	make AMC Concord	price 4,099	mpg 22	rep78 3	headroom 2.5	trunk 11	weight 2,930	length 186

	turn 40	displa~t 121	gear_r~o 3.58	foreign 0

2.	make AMC Pacer	price 4,749	mpg 17	rep78 3	headroom 3.0	trunk 11	weight 3,350	length 173

	turn 40	displa~t 258	gear_r~o 2.53	foreign 0

Here you may find a user-generated facility, `slist`, to be convenient. You can find and install it by typing

```
. findit slist
```

If the variables do not fit on one line, `slist` splits the variables into blocks that do. In the following command, the `id(make)` option lets the identifying variable `make` occur in each block. The `decimal(2)` option lets floating-point numbers be displayed with two decimals. `nolabel` is the default. You can use the `label` option to display labels rather than codes.

```
. slist in 1/2, id(make) decimal(2)
      make            price  mpg  rep78  headroom  trunk  weight  length
1. AMC Concord         4099   22      3      2.50     11    2930     186
2. AMC Pacer           4749   17      3      3.00     11    3350     173
      make            turn  displacement  gear_ratio  foreign
1. AMC Concord          40           121        3.58        0
2. AMC Pacer            40           258        2.53        0
```

browse

The `browse` command lets you see observations and variables in the Data window, much like the `list` command, but `browse` is not good for printing the results:

```
. use lbw1.dta
(Hosmer & Lemeshow data)
. browse id-smoke in 1/5
```

In the Data Browser window, string variables are displayed in red and value labels in blue. Right-clicking in the window lets you toggle between display of codes or value labels.

10.3 Simple tables for categorical variables

`tab1` for one-way tables (frequency tables) and `tab2` for two-way contingency tables (cross tables) are variations of the `tabulate` command. (`tabulate` with one variable creates a frequency table like `tab1`; `tabulate` with two variables creates a cross table like `tab2`.)

tab1

`tab1` (see [R] **tabulate oneway**) creates one-way tables (frequency tables) like the following:

```
. use lbw1.dta
(Hosmer & Lemeshow data)

. tab1 race

-> tabulation of race
       race |      Freq.     Percent        Cum.
------------+-----------------------------------
   1. white |         96       50.79       50.79
   2. black |         26       13.76       64.55
   3. other |         67       35.45      100.00
------------+-----------------------------------
      Total |        189      100.00
```

`tab1` allows you to specify several tables in the varlist, e.g.:

```
. tab1 low race-ftv
```

But beware that if you try to tabulate variables with many different values (like `id` and `bwt`), you get huge but often useless tables.

`tab1` calculates no statistics. Two often-used options are

- `nolabel`, to display codes rather than value labels, and
- `missing`, to include tabulation of missing values. The default is to omit them.

(Continued on next page)

tab2

tab2 (see [R] **tabulate twoway**) creates two-way contingency tables (cross tables) like this:

```
. tab2 low race, column chi2 exact nolog
-> tabulation of low by race
```

```
┌─────────────────────┐
│ Key                 │
├─────────────────────┤
│        frequency    │
│ column percentage   │
└─────────────────────┘
```

birth weight<2500g	race			Total
	1. white	2. black	3. other	
0. No	73	15	42	130
	76.04	57.69	62.69	68.78
1. Yes	23	11	25	59
	23.96	42.31	37.31	31.22
Total	96	26	67	189
	100.00	100.00	100.00	100.00

```
              Pearson chi2(2) =   5.0048   Pr = 0.082
              Fisher's exact =                0.079
```

Some frequently used options are the following:

- column (or col) displays column percent.
- row displays row percent.
- chi2 calculates Pearson's chi-squared test.
- exact calculates Fisher's exact test. nolog restricts the output from the test.
- nolabel displays codes rather than value labels.
- missing includes tabulation of missing values. The default is to omit them.

tab2 does not estimate risk ratios or odds ratios, but you can use cs (section 12.1) to get risk ratios, and cc or tabodds (section 12.2) to get odds ratios.

You can request a three-way table (a two-way table for each value of smoke) by typing

```
. bysort smoke: tab2 low race
```

```
-> smoke = 0. No
```

```
-> tabulation of low by race
```

birthweigh	race			
t<2500g	1. white	2. black	3. other	Total
0. No	40	11	35	86
1. Yes	4	5	20	29
Total	44	16	55	115

```
-> smoke = 1. Yes
```

```
-> tabulation of low by race
```

birthweigh	race			
t<2500g	1. white	2. black	3. other	Total
0. No	33	4	7	44
1. Yes	19	6	5	30
Total	52	10	12	74

tab2 allows you to have many variables in the varlist. The command

```
. tab2 smoke low race
```

gives you 3 two-way tables, one for each possible combination of two variables. But be careful: you can easily produce a huge number of tables. Imagine that you want 10 tables, each of the variables q1–q10 by treatment. With tabulate, you must issue 10 commands to obtain the desired result. If you call tab2 with 11 variables, you get 55 tables — all possible pairs of the 11 variables.

The foreach command (see section 17.4) lets you circumvent the problem:

```
. foreach Q of varlist q1-q10 {
      tab2 'Q' treat
  }
```

The local macro Q is a stand-in for q1 to q10, and the construct generates 10 commands:

```
. tab2 q1 treat
. tab2 q2 treat
. ...
```

(Continued on next page)

proportion

proportion (see [R] **proportion**) estimates proportions with confidence intervals:

```
. proportion race
Proportion estimation                    Number of obs    =      189
        _prop_1: race = 1. white
        _prop_2: race = 2. black
        _prop_3: race = 3. other
```

race	Proportion	Std. Err.	Binomial Wald [95% Conf. Interval]	
_prop_1	.5079365	.0364617	.43601	.5798631
_prop_2	.1375661	.0251212	.0880106	.1871217
_prop_3	.3544974	.034888	.285675	.4233197

With the over() option, you can study subgroups. Here you can see the estimated proportions of smokers and nonsmokers by race:

```
. proportion smoke, over(race)
Proportion estimation                    Number of obs    =      189
        _prop_1: smoke = 0. No
        _prop_2: smoke = 1. Yes
       _subpop_1: race = 1. white
       _subpop_2: race = 2. black
       _subpop_3: race = 3. other
```

Over	Proportion	Std. Err.	Binomial Wald [95% Conf. Interval]	
_prop_1				
_subpop_1	.4583333	.0511205	.3574899	.5591768
_subpop_2	.6153846	.0973009	.4234429	.8073264
_subpop_3	.8208955	.0471982	.7277894	.9140016
_prop_2				
_subpop_1	.5416667	.0511205	.4408232	.6425101
_subpop_2	.3846154	.0973009	.1926736	.5765571
_subpop_3	.1791045	.0471982	.0859984	.2722106

table

`table` is a flexible tool that allows you to build complex tables; see [R] **table**. Here is the same three-way contingency table that we obtained before:

```
. table low race smoke
```

birth weight<2500g	smoked during pregnancy and race					
	0. No			1. Yes		
	1. white	2. black	3. other	1. white	2. black	3. other
0. No	40	11	35	33	4	7
1. Yes	4	5	20	19	6	5

`table` has several options, giving you control over the format of tables. Here the `by()` option organizes the tables for smokers and nonsmokers vertically, `row` and `col` add totals, and `stubwidth()` determines the width of the stub:

```
. table low race, by(smoke) row col stubwidth(20)
```

smoked during pregnancy and birth weight<2500g		race			
		1. white	2. black	3. other	Total
0. No					
	0. No	40	11	35	86
	1. Yes	4	5	20	29
	Total	44	16	55	115
1. Yes					
	0. No	33	4	7	44
	1. Yes	19	6	5	30
	Total	52	10	12	74

Section 10.4 shows you how to use `table` for continuous variables.

tabm

`tabm` is a user-written command that is useful for compact tabulation of several similar categorical variables. It is part of the `tab_chi` package. You can find and install it by typing

```
. findit tabm
```

(Continued on next page)

In `rvary2.dta`, five different raters could rate 10 objects with characters from 1 to 3:

```
. webuse rvary2.dta
. tabm rater*
```

	Values			
Variable	1	2	3	Total
rater1	8	1	1	10
rater2	5	3	2	10
rater3	4	3	2	9
rater4	2	2	4	8
rater5	1	2	7	10
Total	20	11	16	47

groups

`groups` lets you tabulate combinations of several categorical variables. It is a user-written command (Cox 2003b), so you must first install it from the SSC archives (see section 2.2):

```
. ssc install groups
```

Having done that, you can specify the variables to be included:

```
. use lbw1.dta
(Hosmer & Lemeshow data)
. groups low race smoke
```

low	race	smoke	Freq.	Percent
0. No	1. white	0. No	40	21.16
0. No	1. white	1. Yes	33	17.46
0. No	2. black	0. No	11	5.82
0. No	2. black	1. Yes	4	2.12
0. No	3. other	0. No	35	18.52
0. No	3. other	1. Yes	7	3.70
1. Yes	1. white	0. No	4	2.12
1. Yes	1. white	1. Yes	19	10.05
1. Yes	2. black	0. No	5	2.65
1. Yes	2. black	1. Yes	6	3.17
1. Yes	3. other	0. No	20	10.58
1. Yes	3. other	1. Yes	5	2.65

`groups` is a hybrid of a list and a table, and many `list` options apply, such as `sum`, `sepby()`, and `nolabel`.

10.4   Analyzing continuous variables

Description of distributions

For the lbw1.dta dataset, the summarize output (section 10.1) displayed the mean birthweight (bwt) = 2,944 g and SD = 729 g. The detail option gives more information about percentiles, etc. The median (50th percentile) is 2,977 g; the four smallest and the four largest observations are displayed, too:

```
. use lbw1.dta
(Hosmer & Lemeshow data)

. summarize bwt, detail

                       birthweight (grams)

              Percentiles      Smallest
      1%          1021             709
      5%          1790            1021
     10%          1970            1135       Obs                 189
     25%          2414            1330       Sum of Wgt.         189

     50%          2977                       Mean           2944.286
                                 Largest     Std. Dev.      729.016
     75%          3475            4174
     90%          3884            4238       Variance       531464.4
     95%          3997            4593       Skewness      -.2069782
     99%          4593            4990       Kurtosis       2.888821
```

Figure 10.1 is a histogram with the corresponding normal curve (see [R] **histogram**). We made a few extra modifications with this graph (see gph_fig10_1.do, available at this book's web site), but the main command is

```
. histogram bwt, frequency normal
```

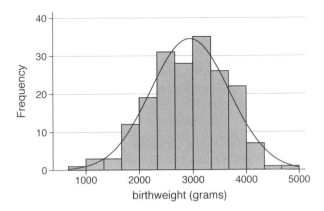

Figure 10.1. Histogram with normal curve

The birthweight distribution does not seem far from a normal distribution. Some people prefer (I do not) to assess agreement with a normal distribution by a so-called Q–Q plot (see figure 10.2 and [R] **diagnostic plots**). The main command for that is

```
. qnorm bwt
```

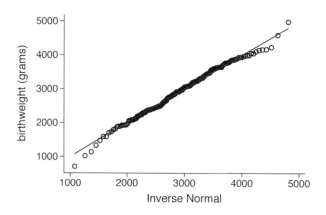

Figure 10.2. Q–Q plot

The conclusion drawn from the Q–Q plot would be the same as that from the histogram, with only minor departures from a normal distribution.

There are also formal tests for departure from a normal distribution, such as the Shapiro–Wilk test (see [R] **swilk**):

```
. swilk bwt
```

		Shapiro-Wilk W test for normal data			
Variable	Obs	W	V	z	Prob>z
bwt	189	0.99263	1.047	0.106	0.45774

The departure from a normal distribution was not at all statistically significant ($Pr = 0.46$). Significance testing for normality may, however, be misleading. With large datasets, even unimportant departures from normality become statistically significant, and the most important tool is visual inspection.

Continuous distributions are often displayed by box-and-whisker plots; see [G] **graph box**. The box displays the interquartile range (the 25th and 75th percentile) and the median. The whiskers display the upper and lower values within 1.5 times the interquartile range beyond the 25th and 75th percentile. Any outliers beyond those limits get their own markers. The main command for the box plot shown in figure 10.3 is

```
. graph box bwt, over(smoke)
```

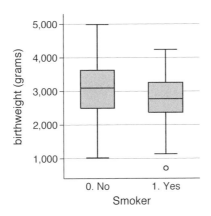

Figure 10.3. Box-and-whisker plot

Transformations

Some analyses, such as *t* tests and linear regression, require the dependent variable to have a normal distribution (conditional on the values of the independent variables), and a transformation may be required to obtain that. gladder (see [R] **ladder**) displays various transformations; the name refers to the "ladder of powers" (Tukey 1977). Figure 10.4 shows an example of the gladder command.

```
. sysuse auto.dta
(1978 Automobile Data)
. gladder mpg, frequency
```

(*Continued on next page*)

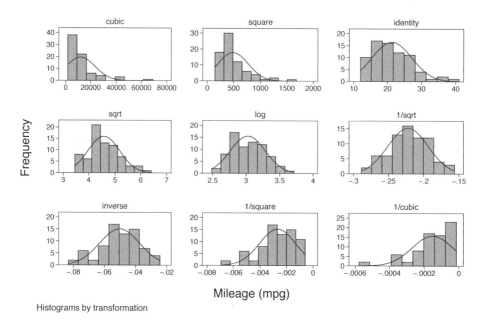

Histograms by transformation

Figure 10.4. gladder displays various transformations

You can obtain a statistical test of normality for the transformations by using ladder:

```
. ladder mpg
```

Transformation	formula	chi2(2)	P(chi2)
cubic	mpg^3	43.59	0.000
square	mpg^2	27.03	0.000
identity	mpg	10.95	0.004
square root	sqrt(mpg)	4.94	0.084
log	log(mpg)	0.87	0.647
1/(square root)	1/sqrt(mpg)	0.20	0.905
inverse	1/mpg	2.36	0.307
1/square	1/(mpg^2)	11.99	0.002
1/cubic	1/(mpg^3)	24.30	0.000

Now you could decide to choose the transformation with the least-significant departure from normality (1/sqrt(mpg)), but you might have a problem in interpreting and communicating it. The inverse (1/mpg) is a better choice because it has a direct interpretation: gas consumption in gallons per mile.

With large datasets, even small and unimportant departures may become significant. Look at the graphs, not the p-values, and consider the interpretability of a transformation.

mean

mean (see [R] **mean**) estimates means. With the over() option, mean displays the mean for subgroups:

```
. use lbw1.dta
(Hosmer & Lemeshow data)

. mean bwt, over(smoke race)

Mean estimation                        Number of obs    =      189

              Over: smoke race
    _subpop_1: 0. No 1. white
    _subpop_2: 0. No 2. black
    _subpop_3: 0. No 3. other
    _subpop_4: 1. Yes 1. white
    _subpop_5: 1. Yes 2. black
    _subpop_6: 1. Yes 3. other

          Over |       Mean    Std. Err.     [95% Conf. Interval]
---------------+-------------------------------------------------
bwt            |
    _subpop_1  |    3428.75    107.0514     3217.574     3639.926
    _subpop_2  |     2854.5    155.3136     2548.119     3160.881
    _subpop_3  |   2814.236    95.50185     2625.843     3002.629
    _subpop_4  |   2827.385    86.90549     2655.949      2998.82
    _subpop_5  |       2504     201.455     2106.597     2901.403
    _subpop_6  |   2757.167    233.8397      2295.88     3218.454
```

tabstat

tabstat (see [R] **tabstat**) displays summary statistics for numeric variables, typically broken down by another variable. You can consider it an extended summarize. In its simplest form, it displays only means:

```
. tabstat age lwt bwt, by(race)

Summary statistics: mean
  by categories of: race (race)

    race |      age        lwt        bwt
---------+-------------------------------
1. white | 24.29167   132.0521    3103.01
2. black | 21.53846   146.8077   2719.692
3. other | 22.38806   120.0299   2804.015
---------+-------------------------------
   Total |  23.2381   129.8201   2944.286
```

(Continued on next page)

`tabstat` offers several summary statistics, listed in table 10.1.

Table 10.1. `tabstat`'s summary statistics

Statistic	Definition	Statistic	Definition
`mean`	Mean	`cv`	Coefficient of variation (`sd/mean`)
`count`	Count of nonmissing	`semean`	Standard error of mean
	observations	`skewness`	Skewness
`n`	Same as count	`kurtosis`	Kurtosis
`sum`	Sum	`p1`	1st percentile
`max`	Maximum	`p5 p10 p25 p50`	5th–50th percentile
`min`	Minimum	`median`	Median (same as p50)
`range`	Range (`max-min`)	`p75 p90 p95 p99`	75th–99th percentile
`sd`	Standard deviation	`iqr`	Interquartile range (`p75-p25`)
`variance`	Variance	`q`	Quartiles (p25 p50 p75)

To display n, mean, sd, cv, semean, and median (or p50) for three variables, type

```
. tabstat age lwt bwt, by(smoke) stat(n mean sd cv semean median)
> longstub

  smoke      stats |      age        lwt        bwt
  0. No          N |      115        115        115
              mean | 23.42609   130.9043   3054.957
                sd | 5.467706   28.41916    752.409
                cv | .2334024   .2170987   .2462912
           se(mean)| .5098662     2.6501    70.1625
               p50 |       23        124       3100

  1. Yes         N |       74         74         74
              mean | 22.94595   128.1351   2772.297
                sd | 5.047424   33.78673   659.8075
                cv | .2199702   .2636805   .2380003
           se(mean)| .5867511   3.927628   76.70106
               p50 |       22        120     2775.5

  Total          N |      189        189        189
              mean |  23.2381   129.8201   2944.286
                sd | 5.298678   30.57515    729.016
                cv | .2280169   .2355194   .2476037
           se(mean)| .3854221   2.224015   53.02811
               p50 |       23        121       2977
```

The `longstub` option shows the name of the statistics in the stub.

You can display the statistics columnwise by using the col(stat) option, and you can control the display format by using the format() option:

```
. tabstat age lwt bwt, stat(n mean sd q) col(stat) format(%8.2f)
```

variable	N	mean	sd	p25	p50	p75
age	189.00	23.24	5.30	19.00	23.00	26.00
lwt	189.00	129.82	30.58	110.00	121.00	140.00
bwt	189.00	2944.29	729.02	2414.00	2977.00	3475.00

tabulate, summarize()

tabulate with the summarize() option (see [R] **tabulate, summarize()**) is similar to tabstat, but it is less flexible. The following command displays a table identical to the table produced by oneway with the tabulate option (see *oneway* later in this section):

```
. tabulate race, summarize(bwt)
```

You can also display the distribution of a continuous variable by two categorical variables:

```
. tabulate race smoke, summarize(bwt)
```

Means, Standard Deviations and Frequencies of birthweight (grams)

race	smoked during pregnancy 0. No	1. Yes	Total
1. white	3428.75 710.09892 44	2827.3846 626.68443 52	3103.0104 727.87244 96
2. black	2854.5 621.25432 16	2504 637.05677 10	2719.6923 638.68388 26
3. other	2814.2364 708.2607 55	2757.1667 810.04465 12	2804.0149 721.30115 67
Total	3054.9565 752.40901 115	2772.2973 659.80748 74	2944.2857 729.01602 189

table

You can use table (see [R] **table**) to build complex tables. In section 10.3, I showed three-way contingency tables; here I only show a simple example of comparing means between subgroups:

```
. table race smoke, contents(mean bwt) format(%9.1f)
```

	smoked during pregnancy	
race	0. No	1. Yes
1. white	3428.8	2827.4
2. black	2854.5	2504.0
3. other	2814.2	2757.2

As you see, there are several partly overlapping possibilities to tabulate means, etc. My favorite is tabstat, which is the most flexible.

oneway

oneway compares means between two or more groups (analysis of variance); see [R] **oneway**.

```
. oneway bwt race, tabulate
```

	Summary of birthweight (grams)		
race	Mean	Std. Dev.	Freq.
1. white	3103.0104	727.87244	96
2. black	2719.6923	638.68388	26
3. other	2804.0149	721.30115	67
Total	2944.2857	729.01602	189

	Analysis of Variance				
Source	SS	df	MS	F	Prob > F
Between groups	5048361.06	2	2524180.53	4.95	0.0081
Within groups	94866937.5	186	510037.298		
Total	99915298.6	188	531464.354		

```
Bartlett's test for equal variances:  chi2(2) =   0.6560  Prob>chi2 = 0.720
```

The descriptive table displays the birthweight distribution (mean and SD) for each race. The ANOVA table tests and rejects (Pr = 0.008) the null hypothesis that there is no difference between means. Among the options are tabulate, which displays a descriptive table, as above, and noanova, which suppresses display of the ANOVA table.

For more complex ANOVAs, see [R] **anova**.

ttest

The family of *t* test commands allows you to compare the means of a normally distributed variable between two groups or to make a paired comparison of two variables; see [R] **ttest**. For example,

```
. ttest bmi, by(sex)                Comparison of two groups; equal variances
                                      assumed
. ttest bmi, by(sex) unequal        Unequal variances (see sdtest)
. ttest prebmi==postbmi             Paired comparison of two variables
. ttest bmidiff==0                  One-sample t test
```

To compare mean birthweights for children born to smoking and nonsmoking mothers:

```
. use lbw1.dta
(Hosmer & Lemeshow data)

. ttest bwt, by(smoke)

Two-sample t test with equal variances
```

Group	Obs	Mean	Std. Err.	Std. Dev.	[95% Conf. Interval]	
0. No	115	3054.957	70.1625	752.409	2915.965	3193.948
1. Yes	74	2772.297	76.70106	659.8075	2619.432	2925.162
combined	189	2944.286	53.02811	729.016	2839.679	3048.892
diff		282.6592	106.9544		71.66693	493.6515

```
    diff = mean(0. No) - mean(1. Yes)                          t =    2.6428
Ho: diff = 0                              degrees of freedom =        187

    Ha: diff < 0                Ha: diff != 0                 Ha: diff > 0
 Pr(T < t) = 0.9955      Pr(|T| > |t|) = 0.0089          Pr(T > t) = 0.0045
```

The middle p-value (Pr $= 0.0089$) is the result of a two-sided test; the smaller of the two others (Pr $= 0.0045$) is the one-sided result.

In [R] **ttest** and the online help, the headings for the various types of t tests can be a bit confusing, with the above two-sample t test having the heading *Two-group mean-comparison test*. The corresponding immediate command has the heading *Two-sample mean-comparison test*, while the paired t test has the heading *Two-sample mean-comparison test (paired)*. Otherwise, the manual's examples are good and illustrative.

sdtest

To test whether the variances (or SDs) can be considered equal, use sdtest (see [R] **sdtest**). To compare SDs between two groups, type

(Continued on next page)

```
. sdtest bwt, by(smoke)
```

Variance ratio test

Group	Obs	Mean	Std. Err.	Std. Dev.	[95% Conf. Interval]
0. No	115	3054.957	70.1625	752.409	2915.965	3193.948
1. Yes	74	2772.297	76.70106	659.8075	2619.432	2925.162
combined	189	2944.286	53.02811	729.016	2839.679	3048.892

```
         ratio = sd(0. No) / sd(1. Yes)                          f =    1.3004
Ho: ratio = 1                                   degrees of freedom =  114, 73

    Ha: ratio < 1                Ha: ratio != 1                 Ha: ratio > 1
  Pr(F < f) = 0.8862         2*Pr(F > f) = 0.2275           Pr(F > f) = 0.1138
```

Again, the middle p-value is the interesting two-sided test $(Pr = 0.23)$, and you can consider the SDs to be equal and use an ordinary t test. You could also have used oneway (see above) and looked at Bartlett's test for equal variances. Regardless of which test you use, be aware that with large datasets even small and unimportant variance differences may be statistically significant.

You can compare the SDs of two variables by typing, for example,

```
. sdtest prebmi==postbmi
```

Despite the similarity with the syntax for a paired t test, sdtest makes an unpaired comparison. A test for paired comparisons, sdpair, is shown in section 15.2.

Nonparametric tests

For an overview of available tests, select

> Help ▷ Search...

and type nonparametric. You will see, for example,

kwallis	Kruskal–Wallis equality-of-populations rank test
signrank	Sign, rank, and median tests (Wilcoxon, Mann–Whitney)

Another good method for searching is to use the menu system; try selecting

> Statistics ▷ Summaries, tables, and tests ▷ Nonparametric tests of hypotheses

One of the options is the Wilcoxon (or Mann–Whitney) rank-sum test. Filling in the dialog to compare birthweight among smoking and nonsmoking mothers, we get

```
. ranksum bwt, by(smoke)
Two-sample Wilcoxon rank-sum (Mann-Whitney) test
        smoke │     obs    rank sum    expected
──────────────┼─────────────────────────────────
        0. No │     115     11915.5       10925
        1. Yes│      74      6039.5        7030
──────────────┼─────────────────────────────────
     combined │     189       17955       17955

unadjusted variance     134741.67
adjustment for ties        -11.98
                        ──────────
adjusted variance       134729.69

Ho: bwt(smoke==0. No) = bwt(smoke==1. Yes)
             z =    2.699
    Prob > |z| =   0.0070
```

Nonparametric tests are based on the ranks rather than the values of the observations, and
you can obtain only p-values, not effect estimates. Also, if the requirements for a parametric test
are fulfilled, the parametric test typically will have better power than its nonparametric cousin.

10.5   Estimating confidence intervals

Many estimating commands display confidence intervals for the estimates. The default is to
use 95% confidence intervals; the level() option is common to many commands and lets you
choose the confidence interval, e.g., 99%:

```
. ttest bwt, by(smoke) level(99)
```

ci

ci lets you calculate confidence intervals for means, proportions, and rates; see [R] **ci**.

To estimate the mean of the continuous variable crea with a 99% confidence interval, type

```
. use ras.dta
(Diagnosis of renal artery stenosis
. ci crea, level(99)
    Variable │      Obs       Mean    Std. Err.     [99% Conf. Interval]
─────────────┼───────────────────────────────────────────────────────────
        crea │      437   93.12815    1.169739      90.10185    96.15444
```

To estimate a proportion with a 95% confidence interval, use the binomial option. The
variable must be coded 0/1:

```
. ci stenosis, binomial

                                              ── Binomial Exact ──
    Variable │      Obs       Mean    Std. Err.    [95% Conf. Interval]
─────────────┼───────────────────────────────────────────────────────────
    stenosis │      437    .228833    .0200952      .1902529    .2711286
```

To estimate a confidence interval for a rate, use the `poisson` option, and state the time-at-risk variable as an argument for the `exposure()` option:

```
. use compliance2.dta
(Compliance data -stset- from randomization)
. ci died, poisson exposure(risktime)
```

Variable	Exposure	Mean	Std. Err.	— Poisson Exact — [95% Conf. Interval]	
died	2634.032	.0391036	.003853	.0319176	.0474244

cii

`cii` is the immediate form of `ci`; see [R] **ci**. You can use the dialogs to produce the results:

```
. db cii
```

The commands have the following formats:

- Normal distribution

```
. cii N mean SD
. cii 372 37.58 16.51
```

Variable	Obs	Mean	Std. Err.	[95% Conf. Interval]	
	372	37.58	.8560036	35.89677	39.26323

- Binomial distribution

```
. cii N events, binomial
. cii 153 40, binomial
```

Variable	Obs	Mean	Std. Err.	— Binomial Exact — [95% Conf. Interval]	
	153	.2614379	.0355248	.1938062	.3385499

The "Mean" column expresses the proportion events (40/153).

- Poisson distribution

```
. cii divisor events, poisson
. cii 2471 40, poisson
```

Variable	Exposure	Mean	Std. Err.	— Poisson Exact — [95% Conf. Interval]	
	2471	.0161878	.0025595	.0115648	.0220432

The divisor ("Exposure") may be a time at risk, in which case "Mean" expresses a rate. With a divisor of 1, you get the Poisson confidence interval for a count.

10.6 Immediate commands

Immediate commands do not use the data in memory. Instead, you enter the data with the command; see [U] **19 Immediate commands**. Typically, you will want to perform some calculations on tabular information. Immediate commands end with i, e.g., `tabi`, `ttesti`, and `cii` (but not all commands that end with i are immediate commands). `cii` was demonstrated in section 10.5. The following sections show the command syntax, but you might prefer to use the dialogs, e.g.,

```
. db tabi
```

tabi

`tabi` is the immediate form of `tab2`, and you can use the same options. Say that you saw table 10.2 in a paper but suspected that the reported $Pr < 0.05$ was misleading because of small numbers.

Table 10.2. Data with suspected misleading $Pr < 0.05$

Treatment	Died	Survived	Total
A	4	10	14
B	7	3	10
Total	11	13	24

$\chi^2 = 4.03$; df $= 1$; $Pr < 0.05$

In `tabi`, you entered the data for each row, separated by \ (backslash):

```
. tabi 4 10 \ 7 3, chi exact
```

```
           |        col
       row |       1          2 |     Total
-----------+--------------------+----------
         1 |       4         10 |        14
         2 |       7          3 |        10
-----------+--------------------+----------
     Total |      11         13 |        24

          Pearson chi2(1) =   4.0328   Pr = 0.045
            Fisher's exact =                0.095
     1-sided Fisher's exact =                0.055
```

Fisher's exact test gave $Pr = 0.095$, so your suspicion was right.

Immediate epitab commands

The immediate `epitab` commands (see [ST] **epitab**) make unstratified analyses only. For help interpreting the output, see sections 12.1, 12.2, and 14.1.

iri is the immediate form of ir (incidence-rate ratio, incidence-rate difference). The arguments must be entered in the correct order, as illustrated in the command below, taking data from table 10.3.

Table 10.3. Incidence-rate data for iri

	Exposed	Unexposed
Events	17	23
Time at risk	231.5	196.4

```
. iri 17 23 231.5 196.4
```

	Exposed	Unexposed		Total		
Cases	17	23		40		
Person-time	231.5	196.4		427.9		
Incidence Rate	.0734341	.1171079		.0934798		
	Point estimate			[95% Conf. Interval]		
Inc. rate diff.	-.0436738			-.1029115	.0155639	
Inc. rate ratio	.6270636			.3144679	1.226403	(exact)
Prev. frac. ex.	.3729364			-.2264033	.6855321	(exact)
Prev. frac. pop	.2017639					

```
                 (midp)   Pr(k<=17) =                     0.0731  (exact)
                 (midp) 2*Pr(k<=17) =                     0.1463  (exact)
```

csi is the immediate form of cs (risk ratio, risk difference). csi is illustrated below, taking data from table 10.4.

Table 10.4. Example data for csi and cci

	Exposed	Unexposed
Event	7	12
No event	19	21

```
. csi 7 12 19 21
```

cci is the immediate form of cc (odds ratio). The arguments are the same as those in csi:

```
. cci 7 12 19 21
```

mcci is the immediate form of mcc for analyzing matched case–control data. It is demonstrated in section 12.2.

ttesti

ttesti is the immediate form of ttest. You input the number of observations, the mean, and the SD for each group. In this example, there are two groups:

```
. ttesti 32 1.35 .27 50 1.77 .33
```

display: Stata as a pocket calculator

The display command gives you the opportunity to perform calculations not involving the data in memory; see [R] **display**. For example,

```
. display 2*c(pi)*7
43.982297
```

You can include explanatory text:

```
. display "The circumference of a circle with radius 7 is " 2*c(pi)*7
The circumference of a circle with radius 7 is 43.982297
```

c(pi) is a Stata constant. c() contains system parameters, settings, and constants; see section 17.1. You can display them by typing

```
. creturn list
```

With display, you can use the built-in functions, e.g., to find a p-value from a chi-squared test:

```
. display chi2tail(1,3.84)
.05004352
```

For more information, see the functions available in [D] **functions**, or type

```
. help functions
```

11 Graphs

Stata's graphics system is powerful. You can often create a desired graph with a simple command or a few clicks in a dialog box; preparing a publication-ready graph may require some more effort. Much of this chapter demonstrates how to create and fine-tune graphs by the command syntax, but section 11.10 illustrates the use of dialogs, and section 11.11 describes the new Graph Editor, which helps you modify an existing graph.

Look at the illustrations in this chapter to get some ideas of the types of graphs available in Stata. At http://www.stata.com/support/faqs/graphics/gph/statagraphs.html, you can find an online tutorial. Also, at http://www.ats.ucla.edu/stat/stata/Library/GraphExamples, you can find a number of graph examples with the commands used. *A Visual Guide to Stata Graphics* (Mitchell 2008) is also accessible and full of examples. For a non-Stata introduction to graph design, I recommend *Creating More Effective Graphs* (Robbins 2005).

The *Graphics Reference Manual* ([G]) has three main sections: Commands, Options, and Styles and concepts. It gives a lot more examples, and it includes the complete documentation of graph commands.

The main graph types described in the *Graphics Reference Manual* are

```
graph bar
graph box
graph dot
graph matrix
graph pie
graph twoway
```

In graph twoway, there are several plot types available, such as twoway scatter and twoway line.

Besides these graph types, there are others (described in [R]) such as histogram and dotplot, and there are graph types related to other topics, such as survival analysis (described in [ST]), e.g., sts graph.

This chapter shows a full do-file for most graphs. Some of the other chapters show graphs, but only with the minimum commands needed to display them in close-to-final form. The full do-files for all graphs are, however, available at this book's web site: http://www.stata-press.com/books/ishr2.html.

11.1   Anatomy of a graph

Figure 11.1 shows the most important elements of a graph. The graph area is the entire figure, including everything in the graph, while the plot area is the central part of the graph, defined by the axes.

A graph consists of several elements: title, legend, axes, and one or more plots, for example, figure 11.1 includes two scatterplots within the same plot area.

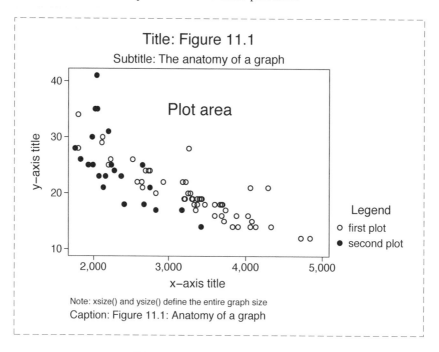

Figure 11.1. Anatomy of a graph

There are two types of elements in a graph like figure 11.1. The plot elements are the dots in the two scatterplots. The graph elements are all the rest: axes, titles, legend, etc. This distinction is reflected in the syntax, as you will see in section 11.2. Below is the do-file that generated figure 11.1. Most elements of this complex command for a complex graph will be explained later.

```
                          ──── gph_fig11_1.do ────
* gph_fig11_1.do

sysuse auto.dta
set scheme lean1

* see section 11.2 for explanation of command listed below
*
twoway                                                            /// G
  (scatter mpg weight if foreign==0)                             /// P
  (scatter mpg weight if foreign==1)                             /// P
  ,                                                               ///
  title("Title: Figure 11.1")                                    /// G
  subtitle("Subtitle: The anatomy of a graph")                   /// G
  ytitle("y-axis title") xtitle("x-axis title")                  /// G
  legend(title("Legend", size(*0.8))                             /// G
    order(1 "first plot" 2 "second plot"))                       /// G
  note("Note: xsize() and ysize() define the entire graph size") /// G
  caption("Caption: Figure 11.1: Anatomy of a graph")            /// G
  text(35 3400 "Plot area", size(*1.5))                          /// G
  graphregion(lpattern(dash) lcolor(black) lwidth(*0.5))         /// G
  xsize(4.4) ysize(3.3)
```

11.2   Anatomy of graph commands

Overall command structure

The general syntax of a graph command is

> [graph] *command* (*plottype*, *plot_options*) (*plottype*, *plot_options*) , *graph_options*

In the command generating figure 11.1, twoway is the graph command, and scatter is a plottype. The syntax above is the syntax style generated by the dialogs, and this book will follow it. You may see another less transparent syntax style, putting bars (| |) where the standard syntax has a right parenthesis closing a plottype specification:

> [graph] *command plottype*, *plot_options* | | *plottype*, *plot_options* | |, *graph_options*

The comma separating the plot specifications from the graph options is important. In the do-file that generates figure 11.1, the P and G comments tell whether a command element is a plot specification or a graph option. In complex commands, I give the pivotal comma a line of its own, just for clarity. (Stata does not care.)

This section will show parts of commands like this:

```
. ..., title("74 car makes")
. twoway (scatter mpg weight, msymbol(Oh)), ...
```

In the first line, `title()` is a graph option; it is preceded by the pivotal comma. In the second line, any graph options can follow after the pivotal comma; `msymbol()` is a plot option, not a graph option.

The full command for a scatterplot is something like

```
. graph twoway (scatter mpg weight), ...
```

It may have this shorter form, which is the syntax generated by the dialogs:

```
. twoway (scatter mpg weight), ...
```

Stata also understands the following short version:

```
. scatter mpg weight
```

Options

Graph commands may have options. As in other Stata commands, a comma precedes the options. `title()` is an option to the `twoway` graph command:

```
. twoway (scatter mpg weight), title("74 car makes")
```

Plottypes may have options. `msymbol()` is an option to `scatter` and is located within the parentheses delimiting the plot specification. `msymbol(Oh)` selects a hollow circle as the marker symbol:

```
. twoway (scatter mpg weight, msymbol(Oh)), ...
```

Options can have suboptions. `size()` is a suboption to the `title()` graph option. Here it sets the title text size to 80% of the default size:

```
. ..., title("74 car makes", size(*0.8))
```

The sequence of options makes no difference.

> Warning: Options, in principle, do not allow a space between the option keyword and its opening parenthesis, like the following (■ denotes a space):
>
> ```
> . ..., title■("74 car makes")
> ```
>
> The error message may be confusing, such as "Unmatched quotes" or "Option not allowed".

> Advice: Graph commands tend to include a lot of nested parentheses, and you may
> make errors (I often do). In the Do-file Editor, you can place the cursor within paren-
> theses and press *Ctrl+B* (B for balance) to see the matching parentheses.

Variable lists: Long and wide data formats

Most two-way plottypes have one or more dependent y variables and one independent x variable, so the scatterplot syntax can be written

> . **twoway (scatter** *yvarlist xvar*, *plot_options*), *graph_options*

The uslifeexp.dta dataset accompanying Stata includes data on U.S. life expectancy for
each year from 1900 to 1999 for the whole nation (le), for males (le_male), for white males
(le_wmale), etc. A graph from these data is shown in section 11.8. See the variables in the
dataset with describe:

```
. sysuse uslifeexp.dta
(U.S. life expectancy, 1900-1999)

. describe

Contains data from C:\Stata\ado\base\u\uslifeexp.dta
  obs:           100                          U.S. life expectancy, 1900-1999
  vars:           10                          30 Mar 2007 04:31
  size:         4,200 (99.9% of memory free)  (_dta has notes)

              storage   display    value
variable name   type    format     label      variable label

year            int     %9.0g                 Year
le              float   %9.0g                 life expectancy
le_male         float   %9.0g                 Life expectancy, males
le_female       float   %9.0g                 Life expectancy, females
le_w            float   %9.0g                 Life expectancy, whites
le_wmale        float   %9.0g                 Life expectancy, white males
le_wfemale      float   %9.0g                 Life expectancy, white females
le_b            float   %9.0g                 Life expectancy, blacks
le_bmale        float   %9.0g                 Life expectancy, black males
le_bfemale      float   %9.0g                 Life expectancy, black females

Sorted by:  year
```

The data structure is "wide". For each observation (a year), there is information on results
for subgroups of the population. For white and black males and females, it looks like this:

```
. list year le_wmale le_wfemale le_bmale le_bfemale if year<1903,
> abbreviate(10)

     year   le_wmale   le_wfemale   le_bmale   le_bfemale

1.   1900       46.6         48.7       32.5         33.5
2.   1901         48           51       32.2         35.3
3.   1902       50.2         53.8       32.9         36.4
```

A corresponding "long" structure would have one observation for each year, sex, and race group. Such a dataset would look like this:

```
. list year le sex race if year<1903, sepby(sex race)
```

```
        | year    le   sex   race |
        |------------------------|
   1.   | 1900  46.6     1      1 |
   2.   | 1901    48     1      1 |
   3.   | 1902  50.2     1      1 |
        |------------------------|
 101.   | 1900  48.7     2      1 |
 102.   | 1901    51     2      1 |
 103.   | 1902  53.8     2      1 |
        |------------------------|
 201.   | 1900  32.5     1      2 |
 202.   | 1901  32.2     1      2 |
 203.   | 1902  32.9     1      2 |
        |------------------------|
 301.   | 1900  33.5     2      2 |
 302.   | 1901  35.3     2      2 |
 303.   | 1902  36.4     2      2 |
```

With a wide data structure, the command to plot a line for each sex and race group is

```
. twoway (line le_wmale le_wfemale le_bmale le_bfemale year), ...
```

With a long data structure, the command gets more complex (best suited for a do-file):

```
. twoway (line le year if sex==1 & race==1)
> (line le year if sex==2 & race==1)
> (line le year if sex==1 & race==2)
> (line le year if sex==2 & race==2)
> , ...
```

In the graph examples, section 11.8, I show examples of both structures. The reshape command (see section 9.6) is a tool for transforming between long and wide data structures.

11.3 Graph size

The twoway scatter command creates scatterplots. Figure 11.2 is the default appearance with the s2mono scheme (for more about schemes, see section 11.4). Here are the commands to produce figure 11.2:

```
. sysuse auto.dta
(1978 Automobile Data)
. set scheme s2mono
. twoway (scatter mpg weight)
```

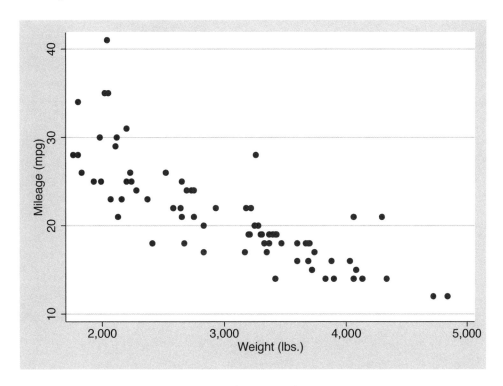

Figure 11.2. Default size of a graph using the s2mono scheme

If you find figure 11.2 too large, you can reduce the size with the xsize() and ysize() graph options, which determine the size of the entire graph area (the arguments are in inches); see figure 11.3.

```
. twoway (scatter mpg weight), xsize(3) ysize(2.2)
```

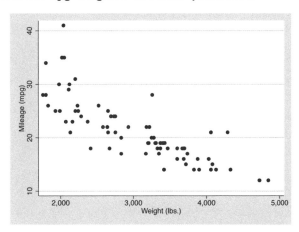

Figure 11.3. Reduced-size graph; marker and text size reduced proportionally

Now the size is right, but the text and marker size shrank with the graph. In particular, the text is too small. To enlarge marker and text size, use the `scale()` graph option. In figure 11.4, text and markers are enlarged by 40% with the following input:

```
. twoway (scatter mpg weight), xsize(3) ysize(2.2) scale(1.4)
```

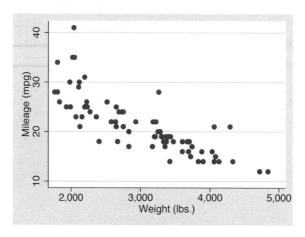

Figure 11.4. Change marker and text size with the `scale()` option

As you will see in section 11.7, you can also modify the size of individual graph and plot elements.

The `xsize()` and `ysize()` options determine the entire graph size, not only the plot area. To control the aspect ratio (the y/x ratio) of the plot area directly, use the `aspectratio()` option. Say that we wanted a square plot area (shown in figure 11.5):

```
. twoway (scatter mpg weight), xsize(3) ysize(2.2) scale(1.4)
> aspectratio(1)
```

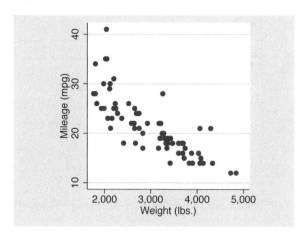

Figure 11.5. Controlling the plot-area aspect ratio with the `aspectratio()` option

11.4 Schemes

Figures 11.2–11.5 used the s2mono scheme with a shaded background and faint grid lines. There are other schemes, such as s1color and s1mono. These schemes have no shaded background and no grid lines, but they have a full frame around the plot area. For example, the following commands produce figure 11.6:

```
. sysuse auto.dta
(1978 Automobile Data)
. set scheme s1mono
. twoway (scatter mpg weight), xsize(3) ysize(2.2) scale(1.4)
```

(Continued on next page)

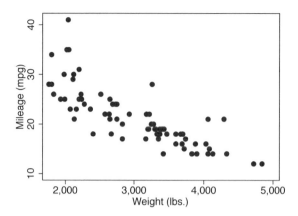

Figure 11.6. s1mono scheme containing a framed plot area, but no grid lines

Two other schemes are lean1 and lean2 (Juul 2003). They avoid colors and grayscales, keeping most things black and white. The lean schemes are not part of official Stata, but you can find and install them by typing

```
. findit lean schemes
```

Style is partly a matter of taste, but it also depends on what you are going to use the graphs for. For a slide show, carefully using colors can be of great value, but colors and grayscales can cause problems when photocopying, and many scientific journals require that you submit lean black and white graphs.

The following commands and figure 11.7 display the same information as figure 11.6 but with the `lean2` scheme:

```
. set scheme lean2
. twoway (scatter mpg weight), xsize(3) ysize(2.2) scale(1.4)
```

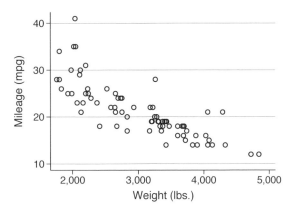

Figure 11.7. Scheme `lean2`

Like `s2color` and `s2mono`, the `lean2` scheme has horizontal grid lines. Like `s1color` and `s1mono`, the `lean1` scheme has no grid lines but has a full frame around the plot area (see figure 11.8):

```
. set scheme lean1
. twoway (scatter mpg weight), xsize(3) ysize(2.2) scale(1.4)
```

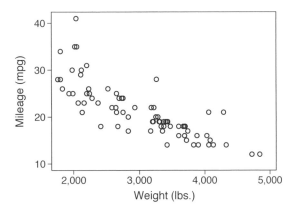

Figure 11.8. Scheme `lean1`

A scheme defines the defaults, but it does not prevent you from making modifications. You might want a blue triangle as a marker (see section 11.7 on marker options):

```
. twoway (scatter mpg weight, msymbol(T) mcolor(blue)), ...
```

or even a triangle with a blue outline and a red fill:

```
. twoway (scatter mpg weight, ms(T) mlcolor(blue) mfcolor(red)), ...
```

To make a scheme (for example, lean1) the default, type

```
. set scheme lean1, permanently
```

To see a list of the schemes installed on your computer, use the command

```
. graph query, schemes
```

A Visual Guide to Stata Graphics (Mitchell 2008) demonstrates several colorful schemes. These schemes may be useful, e.g., for slide shows. To install the schemes, type

```
. net from http://www.stata-press.com/data/vgsg2
. net install vgsg2
```

Read more about schemes in the *Graphics Manual*, starting with [G] **schemes intro**.

11.5   Graph options: Axes

Now things get a bit more complicated. Any command can be given from the command line, but it is easier and safer to build complex commands in do-files; chances are you will need to modify your first attempt. I begin the name of do-files defining graphs with a gph prefix for easy identification, and I begin each do-file with a comment indicating the do-file's name. I also always include a use command (or, as here, a sysuse) to indicate the dataset.

Axis labels, ticks, and grid lines

Stata sets reasonable ticks and labels at the axes, but you can also define them yourself. The following command sets a tick and a label for every 25 years at the x axis. Minor ticks divide each major interval into five intervals. The y-axis label definition had no consequences (see figure 11.9). Stata would have chosen these values anyway. Label specifications follow the rules for numeric lists; see section 4.3.

```
                          ──── gph_fig11_9.do ────
* gph_fig11_9.do

sysuse uslifeexp.dta
set scheme lean2

twoway (line le year)              ///
  ,                                ///
  xlabel(1900(25)2000) xmtick(##5) ///
  ylabel(40(10)80)                 ///
  xsize(3.1) ysize(2.2) scale(1.4)
```

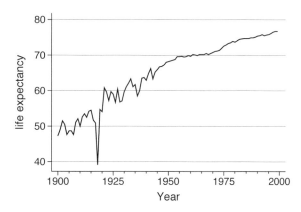

Figure 11.9. Specifying *x*-axis labels and ticks explicitly

You can turn grid lines on and off. The following command in the do-file turns off horizontal and turns on vertical grid lines:

```
                          ──── gph_fig11_10.do ────
* gph_fig11_10.do

sysuse uslifeexp.dta
set scheme lean2

twoway (line le year)              ///
  ,                                ///
  xlabel(1900(20)2000, grid)       ///
  ylabel(, nogrid)                 ///
  xsize(3.1) ysize(2.2) scale(1.4)
```

Figure 11.10 shows the graph resulting from the above do-file.

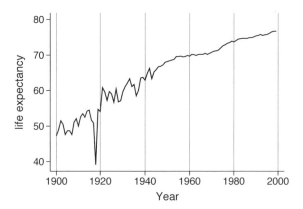

Figure 11.10. Turning horizontal grid lines off and vertical grid lines on

By definition, the axes in twoway graphs are continuous, but categorical variables may be used. To display value labels rather than codes, use the valuelabel suboption (the ticks were turned off, too):

    . ..., xlabel(1(1)8, valuelabel noticks)

Tick labels can also be specified explicitly in the label option. If you want to include a leading zero in the y-axis labels, like in figure 11.11, use the ylabel() option:

    . ..., ylabel(.1 "0.1" .2 "0.2" .5 "0.5" 1 10 ...)

In the s1 and s2 schemes, the y-axis labels by default are vertically oriented. If you want horizontal y-axis labels (as in the lean schemes) with an s1 or s2 scheme, type

    . ..., ylabel(, angle(0))

To remove labels and ticks from the x axis, type

    . ..., xlabel(none)

To hide the y axis, use

    . ..., yscale(off)

You can expand an axis beyond what the data require by defining a value range:

    . ..., xscale(range(0.5 8.5))

Most graphs by default leave some space (the plot-region margin) between axes and the closest plot values, but in figure 11.11, we want the x axis to start at zero. You can do this by using the plotregion(margin(l=0)) option (l for left, r for right, t for top, b for bottom). If you want all margins to be zero, the option is plotregion(margin(zero)).

If you want to display decimal commas rather than periods, use the Stata command

```
. set dp comma
```

and return to the default decimal period by typing

```
. set dp period
```

Log-scaled axes

You can use log scales, but a detailed axis-label specification is often required, as in figure 11.11. By default, there would be too many horizontal grid lines. In the do-file below, the lines were turned off by `ylabel()`'s `nogrid` option, and four thin reference lines were drawn by `yline()` instead to produce figure 11.11.

```
───────────────────── gph_fig11_11.do ─────────────────────
* gph_fig11_11.do

cd C:\docs\ishr2
use agemort.dta
set scheme lean2

twoway (line mort age)                                   ///
  ,                                                      ///
  plotregion(margin(l=0))                                ///
  yscale(log)                                            ///
  ylabel(.1 "0.1" .2 "0.2" .5 "0.5" 1 2 5 10            ///
       20 50 100 200 500, nogrid)                        ///
  yline(0.1 1 10 100, lwidth(*0.5))                      ///
  xsize(3.1) ysize(2.2) scale(1.4)
```

(*Continued on next page*)

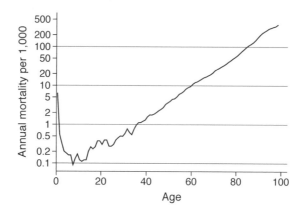

Figure 11.11. Log-scaled y axis

In figure 11.11, there are probably too many y-axis labels. The following do-file (which produces figure 11.12) shows another way to put labels and ticks on a log-scaled axis, by using `ymticks()` (minor ticks):

```
                           ───── gph_fig11_12.do ─────
* gph_fig11_12.do

cd C:\docs\ishr2
use agemort.dta
set scheme lean2

twoway (line mort age)                               ///
  ,                                                  ///
  plotregion(margin(l=0))                            ///
  yscale(log)                                        ///
  ylabel(.1 "0.1" 1 10 100)                          ///
  ymticks(.2(.1).9  2(1)9  20(10)90  200(100)500)    ///
  xsize(3.1) ysize(2.2) scale(1.4)
```

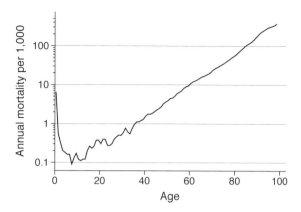

Figure 11.12. Log-scaled y axis; alternative labeling

Multiple axes

You can have more than one x and one y axis. The following do-file produces figure 11.13, reconstructed from Doll and Hill (1950). Figure 11.13 has two y axes, one for lung cancer mortality and one for cigarette consumption. The original information about pounds of tobacco was recalculated to grams (1 cigarette = 1 g).

(Continued on next page)

```
───────── gph_fig11_13.do ─────────
* gph_fig11_13.do

set scheme lean1

clear
input year tobacco cancer
1900  .4    .5
1907  .7    .6
1912  .9   1.0
1924 1.9   1.9
1930 2.4   4.0
1936 2.8   7.5
1947 4.2  22.5
end

generate cigarettes = 454*tobacco        // (1 lb. = 454 grams)

twoway                                                          ///
  (line cancer year, yaxis(1) lpattern(1))                     ///
  (line cigarettes year, yaxis(2) lpattern(dash))              ///
  ,                                                            ///
  xtitle("Year")                                               ///
  ytitle("Annual lung cancer" "mortality per 100,000", axis(1)) ///
  ytitle("Cigarettes per person per year", axis(2))            ///
  legend(order(2 "Cigarette consumption" 1 "Lung cancer mortality")) ///
  plotregion(margin(b=0))                                      ///
  xsize(5) ysize(2) aspectratio(0.75) scale(1.4)
```

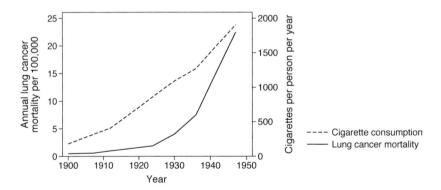

Figure 11.13. Graph with two y axes

In the plot specifications, the axes are referred to as yaxis(1) and yaxis(2). In the ytitle() options, they are referred to as axis(1) and axis(2).

11.6   Graph options: Text elements

Titles and texts

Graph title and subtitle, axis titles, notes, and captions are defined as shown in figure 11.1. By default, axis titles use variable labels if they are defined, otherwise they use variable names.

You can define a two-line text, as in figure 11.13, by splitting up the text in quotes. For example,

```
. ..., ytitle("Annual lung cancer" "mortality per 100,000")
```

Legends

Say that we want to put two scatterplots — one for domestic and one for foreign cars — in one graph (see figure 11.14). We start with the s1mono scheme:

```
──────────────────── gph_fig11_14.do ────────────────────
* gph_fig11_14.do

sysuse auto.dta
set scheme s1mono

twoway                                      ///
  (scatter mpg weight if foreign==0)        ///
  (scatter mpg weight if foreign==1)        ///
  ,                                         ///
  xsize(3.1) ysize(2.2) scale(1.4)
```

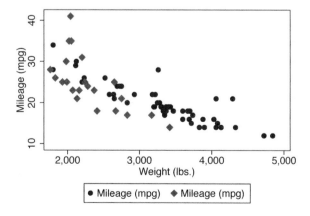

Figure 11.14. Two plots in one graph

If there is more than one plot in a graph, the legend is used to explain the meaning of the various marker and line styles. In figure 11.14, the legend does not display the information we need. To get the right information, we must include a `legend()` option in the `twoway` command.

We might also find that the two gray-scaled symbols in figure 11.14 are too indistinct. One option is to define the symbols explicitly (see section 11.7), and another option is to see what the `lean` schemes do. We also put a title for the legend in figure 11.15:

```
_____ gph_fig11_15.do _____
* gph_fig11_15.do

sysuse auto.dta
set scheme lean1

twoway                                                       ///
  (scatter mpg weight if foreign==0)                         ///
  (scatter mpg weight if foreign==1)                         ///
  ,                                                          ///
  legend(title("Origin") order(1 "Domestic" 2 "Foreign")) ///
  xsize(3.1) ysize(2.2) scale(1.4)
```

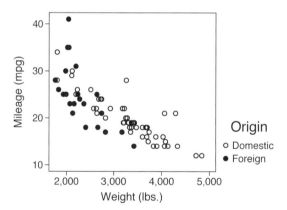

Figure 11.15. `lean` schemes provide distinct markers, but legend placement distorts plot area

We now see more distinct symbols, but the graph became distorted — why? Whereas the `s1` and `s2` schemes put the legend below the x axis, the `lean` schemes put it to the right of the plot area. The `xsize()` and `ysize()` options define the size of the entire graph, including axis titles, labels, and the legend. To compensate, `xsize()` must be increased. In this next example, 3.8 inches seems to work. We also reduce the size of the legend title (see figure 11.16):

```
────────────────── gph_fig11_16.do ──────────────
* gph_fig11_16.do

sysuse auto.dta
set scheme lean1

twoway                                      ///
  (scatter mpg weight if foreign==0)        ///
  (scatter mpg weight if foreign==1)        ///
  ,                                         ///
  legend(title("Origin", size(*0.8))        ///
    order(1 "Domestic" 2 "Foreign"))        ///
  xsize(3.8) ysize(2.2) scale(1.4)
```

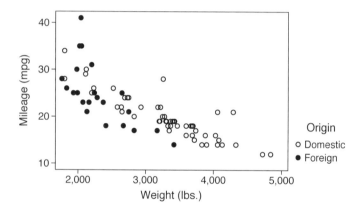

Figure 11.16. Distorted plot area corrected by increasing xsize()

Instead of experimenting with xsize() and ysize() to obtain the desired plot aspect ratio, you can use the aspectratio() option. Be generous with the xsize() option, and use aspectratio() to control the y/x ratio of the plot area (it looks exactly like figure 11.16):

```
. ..., xsize(4) ysize(2.2) scale(1.4) aspectratio(0.7)
```

Placing text elements

The placement of text elements, such as titles and the legend, is defined by location relative to the plot area (ring position) and a direction (clock position); see [G] **title_options**. The placement of elements in our anatomy of a graph (figure 11.1) was determined by the scheme applied (lean1); the placements are shown in table 11.1. The only difference from the s1 and s2 schemes is the legend placement; s1 and s2 put the legend at pos(6).

Table 11.1. Placement of text elements with the lean schemes

Element	Ring position ring()	Clock position pos()	Position can be modified?
Plot area	0	...	No
y-axis title	1	9	No
x-axis title	1	6	No
Title	7	12	Yes
Subtitle	6	12	Yes
Legend	3	4	Yes
Note	4	7	Yes
Caption	5	7	Yes

The details of the outer rings are hardly interesting to most users, but specifying ring(0) places an object within the plot area. To place the legend in the upper-right corner, specify the two o'clock position with pos(2) (see figure 11.17):

```
————————————————— gph_fig11_17.do ——————————————
* gph_fig11_17.do

sysuse auto.dta
set scheme lean1

twoway                                                      ///
  (scatter mpg weight if foreign==0)                        ///
  (scatter mpg weight if foreign==1)                        ///
  ,                                                         ///
  legend(order(1 "Domestic" 2 "Foreign") ring(0) pos(2))   ///
  xsize(3.1) ysize(2.2) scale(1.4)
```

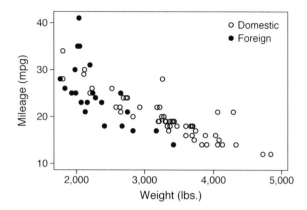

Figure 11.17. Legend placed inside plot area by using the `ring(0)` argument

You can put a text block anywhere in the plot area (see the example in figure 11.1) by specifying its y and x coordinates. `place(0)` (the default) means that the coordinates apply to the center of the text block. `place(8)` means that the text is placed at eight o'clock, relative to the point defined by the coordinates. `place(sw)` means the same as `place(8)`.

```
. ..., text(35 3400 "Plot area", place(0))
```

Because `place(0)` is the default, this suboption could have been omitted.

11.7 Plot options: Markers, lines, etc.

Stata chooses markers, line styles, etc., from a style list, which depends on the scheme selected. I recommend that you run the first version of a graph command without specifying marker or line options and then modify them, if you need to do that.

Table 11.2 shows the options for markers, bars, and lines. Examples of their use are shown in the following subsections.

(Continued on next page)

Table 11.2. Options for defining the appearance of lines, bars, markers, etc.

All elements, except markers		Markers	
Overall color:	color()	Overall color:	mcolor()
Fill color:	fcolor()	Fill color:	mfcolor()
Line, outline color:	lcolor()	Outline color:	mlcolor()
Line, outline width:	lwidth()	Outline width:	mlwidth()
Line, outline pattern:	lpattern()	Marker symbol:	msymbol()
		Marker size:	msize()

Bars, areas, textboxes, etc., have an outline and a fill that can be defined separately, e.g., by using lcolor() to specify the outline color and fcolor() to specify the fill color. Marker options all start with m; for example, mlcolor() defines the marker outline color, and mfcolor() the marker fill color.

Colors

To see a list of the colors available, use the command

```
. help colorstyle
```

To see one color, e.g., lavender, on the screen, type

```
. palette color lavender
```

If you installed the schemes related to *A Visual Guide to Stata Graphics* (see section 11.4), the following command will display a full color palette:

```
. vgcolormap
```

Gray colors have names from gs0 (black) to gs16 (white).

```
. ..., bar(3, fcolor(gs9))
```

When printing or photocopying graphs with colors or gray scales, look carefully at the result. The appearance is sensitive to printer setup, toner quality, etc. For more on this topic, see section 11.12.

Lines

You can see most of the available line patterns by typing

```
. palette linepalette
```

Figure 11.18 shows a modified palette of the patterns.

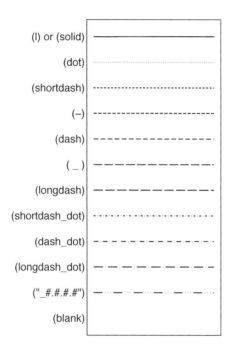

Figure 11.18. Line patterns

Besides using the patterns created by Stata, you can create your own by using a formula, e.g,

```
. twoway (line le year, lpattern("_#.#.#.#")), ...
```

where # puts a little extra space between the elements.

The main use of line patterns is to connect line plots (the `lpattern()` option), but you can also use it for, e.g., bar outlines.

(Continued on next page)

Marker symbols

Figure 11.19 shows the marker symbols used for scatterplots, etc. To create it, type

```
. palette symbolpalette
```

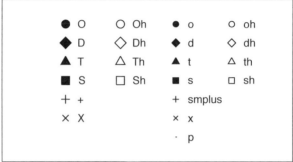

(symbols shown at larger than default size)

Figure 11.19. Marker symbols

To define a hollow circle, type, for example,

```
. twoway (scatter mpg weight, msymbol(Oh)), ...
```

A hollow circle (Oh) is transparent. You can obtain a circle with a nontransparent white fill by typing, for example,

```
. twoway (scatter mpg weight, msymbol(O) mfcolor(white)), ...
```

A scheme has a default sequence of markers. The s1 and s2 schemes also vary the marker colors, whereas the lean schemes keep all markers black. A scheme defines the defaults, but it does not prevent you from making modifications. You might want a blue triangle as the marker in our example:

```
. twoway (scatter mpg weight, msymbol(T) mcolor(blue)), ...
```

Or maybe you want a triangle with a blue outline and a red fill:

```
. twoway (scatter mpg weight, ms(T) mlcolor(blue) mfcolor(red)), ...
```

Modifying size of elements

The width of a line is controlled by the `lwidth()` option, as in

```
. twoway (line le year, lpattern(dash) lwidth(*0.8)), ...
```

making the line width 80% of the default.

The size of a marker is controlled by the `msize()` option, as in

```
. twoway (scatter mpg weight, msymbol(Th) msize(*1.5)), ...
```

making the marker size 50% larger than the default.

As shown in section 11.3, the `scale()` option lets you modify the size of many elements at once (e.g., text, symbol sizes).

11.8   Graph examples

Here you will find illustrations of some important graph types, including the commands that generated the graphs. The appearance is different from the manual's graphs; it comes from the schemes `lean1` and `lean2`, described in section 11.4.

I will show the do-file used to make each graph, including the data for the graph or a `use` command. I suggest giving do-files that generate graphs a gph prefix for easy identification.

Histograms

A histogram illustrates the distribution of a continuous variable; see [R] **histogram**. Figure 11.20 shows the weight distribution of 74 car makes. If you do not specify the number of bars (or number of bins, as it is often called in a histogram context), the placement of the first bar, or the width of bars, Stata will decide for you:

```
─────────────────────── gph_fig11_20.do ───────────────────────
* gph_fig11_20.do

sysuse auto.dta
set scheme lean2

histogram weight, xsize(3.1) ysize(2.2) scale(1.4)
```

(Continued on next page)

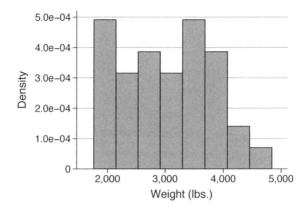

Figure 11.20. Histogram

The look of figure 11.20 is not quite satisfactory, so let's make some modifications: We want to have bars reflect "natural" 500-pound groups (the start() and width() options). The y axis displays the density; we want the number of observations (the frequency option). We also want a normal curve and a kernel density curve overlaid (the normal and kdensity options). Our modifications to this do-file produce figure 11.21.

```
───────────────── gph_fig11_21.do ─────────────────
* gph_fig11_21.do

sysuse auto.dta
set scheme lean2

histogram weight               ///
   ,                           ///
   frequency                   ///
   normal                      ///
   kdensity                    ///
   start(1000) width(500)      ///
   xsize(3.1) ysize(2.2) scale(1.4)
```

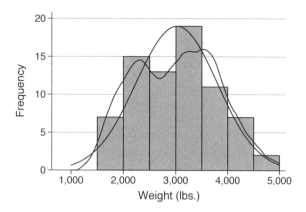

Figure 11.21. Histogram with a normal and a kernel density curve overlaid

It is striking that the shapes of the histograms in figure 11.20 and 11.21 are so different. With few observations, varying the cutpoints between bins can make quite a difference in appearance. The kernel density curve can be considered a smoothed version of a histogram (for more information, see [R] **kdensity**). Here it suggests that the cars consist of two subpopulations, which is actually the case.

Box plots and dot plots

In a box-and-whisker plot, the box displays the interquartile range (the 25th–75th percentiles) and the median (see [G] **graph box**). The whiskers display the upper and lower values within 1.5 times the interquartile range beyond the 25th and 75th percentile. Any outliers beyond that get their own marker. In figure 11.22, the orientation is horizontal and is obtained by the graph hbox command; graph box gives a vertical orientation. The value labels in figure 11.22 are less than optimal. For the over() option, see *Bar graphs* later in this section.

```
                        ─────── gph_fig11_22.do ───────
* gph_fig11_22.do

cd C:\docs\ishr2
use lbw1.dta
set scheme lean2

graph hbox bwt                  ///
    ,                           ///
    over(smoke) over(race)      ///
    xsize(3.8) ysize(2.2) scale(1.4)
```

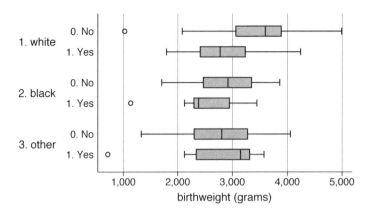

Figure 11.22. Horizontal box plot

A dot plot can be used for similar purposes. It can be considered a kind of histogram, and it is described in the *Base Reference Manual* (see [R] **dotplot**). It is different from the plottype described in [G] **graph dot**. In the following do-file (which produces figure 11.23), the center option makes the columns symmetrical, the nx() option sets the horizontal dot density, and the ny() option sets the number of bins. You might need to experiment to get a satisfactory result. msymbol(O) defines the marker symbol as a filled circle.

```
──────────────────────── gph_fig11_23.do ────────────────────────
* gph_fig11_23.do

sysuse auto.dta
set scheme lean1

dotplot weight                      ///
    ,                               ///
    over(foreign) center msymbol(O) ///
    nx(14) ny(20)                   ///
    xsize(2.8) ysize(2.2) scale(1.4)
```

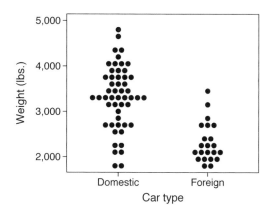

Figure 11.23. Dot plot

Bar graphs

Bar graphs typically show the distribution of a quantity (count, sum, mean) over groups defined by one or more categorical variables; see [G] **graph bar**.

The main elements in the graph bar command are

> . **graph bar** (*stat*) *yvarlist* [(*stat*) *yvarlist*]**,** **over**(*xvar*) [**over**(*xvar*)]
> *other_options*

(*stat*) can be any of the statistics available in collapse; see [D] **collapse** or type

> . **help collapse**

(*stat*) can be, e.g.,

(asis)   the values as they are (one observation per group, as in figure 11.24)
(mean)   mean of values in a group (the default)
(count)   number of valid observations in a group

The over() option defines the groups to be displayed. The graph hbar command gives horizontal bars.

Figure 11.24 illustrates the prevalence of diabetes. Data are entered in wide form in the do-file:

(Continued on next page)

```
———————————— gph_fig11_24.do ————————————
* gph_fig11_24.do

clear
input str5 age diabm diabf
16-24    .9    .2
25-44    .8    .8
45-66   3.8   2.9
67-79   8.2   5.4
80+      9.1   7.2
end

set scheme lean2

graph bar (asis) diabm diabf              ///
  ,                                       ///
  over(age)                               ///
  b1title("Age")                          ///
  ytitle("Prevalence (percent)")          ///
  legend(order(1 "Males" 2 "Females"))    ///
  blabel(bar, format(%03.1f))             ///
  xsize(4.4) ysize(2.2) scale(1.4)
```

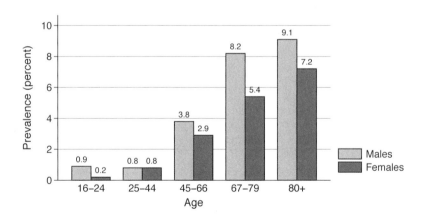

Figure 11.24. Bar graph constructed from tabular data

There are two *y* variables in the *yvarlist* (diabm and diabf). The statistic (asis) corresponds to one observation per group. The default statistic is (mean), and with one observation per group, a value and its mean are the same. The command could have been

```
. graph bar (mean) diabm diabf, ...
```

or even, since (`mean`) is the default statistic,

```
. graph bar diabm diabf, ...
```

For some reason, the `xtitle()` option is not valid for bar graphs. To generate an x-axis title, you can, however, use `b1title()` instead.

The `blabel()` option lets you put labels on top of the bars. `format(%03.1f)` displays leading zeros. Actually, I prefer to avoid such labels, but now you know how to make them.

Bar fill colors (see table 11.2) are assigned automatically according to the scheme. The following option would generate a dark fill for females:

```
. ..., bar(2, fcolor(gs3))
```

The `lbw1.dta` dataset is in long format. The `over()` option can be nested to three layers. This do-file produces figure 11.25, which has two layers:

```
──────────────────── gph_fig11_25.do ────────────────────
* gph_fig11_25.do

cd C:\docs\ishr2
use lbw1.dta
set scheme lean2

graph bar (mean) bwt              ///
  ,                               ///
  over(smoke) over(race)          ///
  xsize(3.3) ysize(2.2) scale(1.4)
```

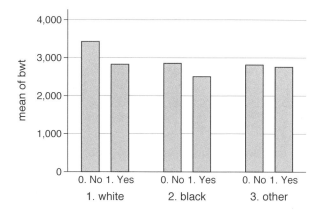

Figure 11.25. Bar graph nested to two layers

The bars are labeled according to the value labels in the dataset. They are, however, poor labels, and I must redefine the value labels before using the `graph` command.

Figure 11.26 shows improved titles and labels. It also shows how the `asyvars` option can be used to restructure the graph: it behaves as if the data were in wide format with two y variables (birthweight among smokers and nonsmokers) and the command had one `over()` option. Here is the do-file:

```
——————————————————— gph_fig11_26.do ———————————
* gph_fig11_26.do

cd C:\docs\ishr2
use lbw1.dta
set scheme lean2

label define smoke 0 "Nonsmokers" 1 "Smokers", modify
label values smoke smoke
label define race 1 "Whites" 2 "Blacks" 3 "Others", modify

graph bar (mean) bwt                    ///
  ,                                     ///
  over(smoke) over(race) asyvars        ///
  ytitle("Mean birthweight (grams)")    ///
  xsize(3.9) ysize(2.2) scale(1.4)
```

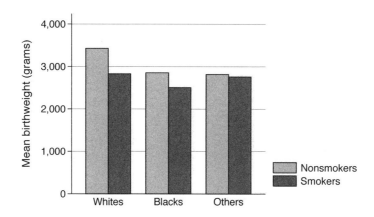

Figure 11.26. Bar graph using the `asyvars` option to restructure the graph

When comparing the distribution between groups of an ordinal (rank-ordered) variable, stacked bars are efficient. In figure 11.27, the repair records of domestic and foreign cars are compared (1 is a poor and 5 a good record). In this graph, the relative bar heights should reflect the number of cars, hence the (`count`) statistic. I could have counted any variable, as long as I was sure that it had no missing values. I chose the safe way and created the help variable `x`. The use of a consistent light–dark gradient and the `order()` suboption to the `legend()` option ensures that the legend order corresponds to the order in the bars. Here is the do-file:

```
———————————————— gph_fig11_27.do ————————————————
* gph_fig11_27.do

sysuse auto.dta
set scheme lean2
generate x=1
graph bar (count) x                          ///
   ,                                         ///
   over(rep78) over(foreign)                 ///
   asyvars percent stack                     ///
   bar(1, fcolor(gs0))                       ///
   bar(2, fcolor(gs6))                       ///
   bar(3, fcolor(gs10))                      ///
   bar(4, fcolor(gs13))                      ///
   bar(5, fcolor(gs16))                      ///
   legend(title("Repair" "record", size(*0.8))  ///
     order(5 4 3 2 1))                       ///
   ytitle("Percent")                         ///
   b1title("Origin")                         ///
   xsize(2.8) ysize(2.2) scale(1.4)
```

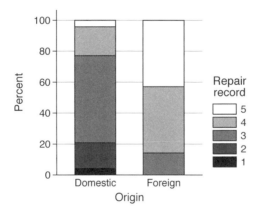

Figure 11.27. Stacked bars

Scatterplots

You have seen several scatterplots already. Markers are defined by symbol (msymbol()); size (msize()); overall color (mcolor()); or outline color (mlcolor()) and fill color (mfcolor()); see table 11.2 and figure 11.19.

To define a hollow circle, type, for example,

```
. twoway (scatter mpg weight, msymbol(Oh)), ...
```

A hollow circle (Oh) is transparent. You can obtain a circle with a nontransparent white fill by typing, for example,

```
. twoway (scatter mpg weight, msymbol(O) mfcolor(white)), ...
```

The following do-file produces figure 11.28, which displays enlarged hollow triangles (Th) and small filled diamonds (d) as markers:

```
──────────────────────── gph_fig11_28.do ────────────────────────
* gph_fig11_28.do

sysuse auto.dta
set scheme lean1

twoway                                                              ///
  (scatter mpg weight if foreign==0, msymbol(Th) msize(*1.5))  ///
  (scatter mpg weight if foreign==1, msymbol(d))               ///
  ,                                                                ///
  legend(order(1 "Domestic" 2 "Foreign"))                        ///
  xsize(3.8) ysize(2.2) scale(1.4)
```

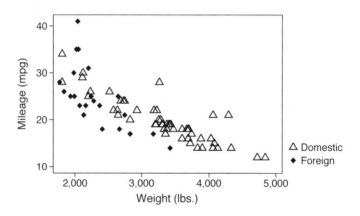

Figure 11.28. Scatterplot using explicitly defined markers

The markers in a scatterplot can be weighted; that is, they can vary in size according to a third variable (see figure 11.29). The census.dta dataset includes demographic information for the 50 United States. In the next do-file, we calculate urban, the degree of urbanization, and examine the relationship between urbanization and median age (medage). Each state is represented by a circle whose area is proportional to the population size (pop). I had to try a few times before I found a reasonable marker size (the msize() plot option). For information about weighting, see section 4.5.

```
                        ———————— gph_fig11_29.do ————————
* gph_fig11_29.do

sysuse census.dta
generate urban = 100*popurban/pop
label variable urban "Urbanization (percent)"
format medage %9.0g
set scheme lean1

twoway                                                           ///
  (scatter medage urban [fweight=pop], msymbol(Oh) msize(*0.5))  ///
  ,                                                              ///
  yscale(range(24 35))                                           ///
  xlabel(30(10)100)                                              ///
  note("The marker for each state is proportional to population size") ///
  xsize(2.9) ysize(2.2) scale(1.4)
```

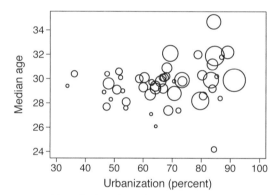

The marker for each state is proportional to population size

Figure 11.29. Weighted scatterplot

A linear regression line (see [G] **graph twoway lfit** and [G] **graph twoway lfitci**), a quadratic regression line (see [G] **graph twoway qfit** and [G] **graph twoway qfitci**), a smoothed lowess curve (see [G] **graph twoway lowess**), or a smoothed kernel-weighted local polynomial curve (see [G] **graph twoway lpoly** and [G] **graph twoway lpolyci**) can be overlaid on a scatterplot.

Line plots

Connecting lines are used in the twoway line and twoway connected commands; for details, see [G] **graph twoway line** and [G] **graph twoway connected**. Lines are defined by lpattern(), lcolor(), and lwidth(); see table 11.2. Figure 11.18 shows the line patterns available.

In figure 11.30, we use the data about U.S. life expectancy to plot the life expectancy for white and black males and females. The data are in wide format, as described in section 11.2. Each observation includes information on the independent variable (year) and the four dependent variables (le_wmale, le_wfemale, le_bmale, le_bfemale). A scheme has a default sequence of line patterns to be used. I chose lean2 as the scheme. The data are sorted by year; if they had not been, the result would be nonsense. The first command is rather short, but I guess it will need modifications, so I use a do-file:

```
——————————————— gph_fig11_30.do ———————————————
* gph_fig11_30.do

sysuse uslifeexp.dta
set scheme lean2

twoway                                                      ///
   (line le_wmale le_wfemale le_bmale le_bfemale year) ///
   ,                                                        ///
   xsize(4.4) ysize(2.2) scale(1.4)
```

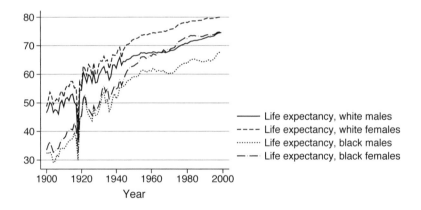

Figure 11.30. Four line plots in one plot area with default line styles and legend

Figure 11.30 can be improved. In the following do-file, which displays figure 11.31, I chose thin lines for whites and dashed lines for males. This graph has four line plots representing four different dependent variables. In the lpattern() and lwidth() options, I specified the line pattern and width for all four lines in the sequence they were mentioned in the line plot specification. In the legend() option, I chose an order corresponding to the overall sequence in the graph:

```
―――――――――――――――――――――――――― gph_fig11_31.do ――――――――――――――――――――――
* gph_fig11_31.do

sysuse uslifeexp.dta
set scheme lean2

twoway                                                    ///
  (line le_wmale le_wfemale le_bmale le_bfemale year,  ///
    lpattern(dash l dash l) lwidth(*.8 *.8 *1.4 *1.4)) ///
  ,                                                       ///
  ytitle("Life expectancy")                             ///
  legend(order(2 "White females" 1 "White males"        ///
    4 "Black females" 3 "Black males"))                 ///
  xsize(4.4) ysize(2.2) scale(1.4)
```

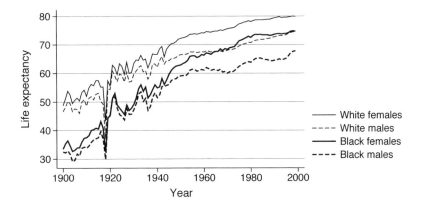

Figure 11.31. Line styles, legend text, and legend order specified explicitly

A twoway connected plot is a combined line plot and scatterplot. Figure 11.32 displays the results of a study using the SF-36 questionnaire of health-related quality of life among 140 patients (obs), compared with the expected from population norm data (norm). There were a few missing values, so no scale had 140 valid observations. Here is the do-file:

(Continued on next page)

─────────────────────── gph_fig11_32.do ───────────────────────

```
* gph_fig11_32.do

clear
input scale n obs sd norm
1 139 60.810 27.346 70.77
2 139 37.650 42.056 62.01
3 136 59.397 28.568 73.66
4 139 57.647 21.686 66.27
5 138 52.754 25.553 64.24
6 137 76.642 26.810 85.85
7 138 51.691 41.869 73.59
8 139 73.065 21.538 79.99
end

generate se=sd/sqrt(n)
generate ci1=obs+1.96*se
generate ci2=obs-1.96*se

label define scale 1 "PF" 2 "RP" 3 "BP" 4 "GH" 5 "VT" 6 "SF" 7 "RE" 8 "MH"
label values scale scale

set scheme lean1

twoway                                                         ///
  (connected obs scale, msymbol(O) lpattern(l))               ///
  (connected norm scale, msymbol(O) mfcolor(white) lpattern(dash)) ///
  (rcap ci1 ci2 scale)                                        ///
  ,                                                           ///
  ytitle("Mean score")                                        ///
  xtitle("SF-36 subscale")                                    ///
  xlabel(1(1)8, valuelabel noticks)                           ///
  xscale(range(0.5 8.5))                                      ///
  legend(order(2 "Expected" 1 "Observed" 3 "95% CI"))         ///
  xsize(3.9) ysize(2.2) scale(1.4)
```

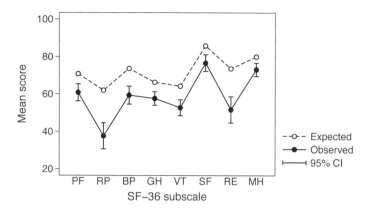

Figure 11.32. Two `connected` and one `rcap` plot

Figure 11.32 includes three plots: two `connected` and one `rcap`. In two-way plots, both axes are continuous, so you could not have a categorical variable (PF, RP, etc.) on the x axis. The solution is to use a numerical variable and use value labels to indicate the meaning. This graph style is often used to present SF-36 results, although connecting lines may be illogical when displaying eight qualitatively different scales.

For the expected values, I chose a marker with a white fill. With a hollow marker (Oh), the connecting line would have been visible within the marker.

The x-axis labels could also have been defined within the `xlabel()` option:

```
 . ... , xlabel(1 "PF" 2 "RP" 3 "BP" 4 "GH" 5 "VT" 6 "SF" 7 "RE" 8 "MH")
```

`xscale(range(0.5 8.5))` made the x axis wider than required by the data to increase the distance between the plot symbols and the plot margin.

`rcap` is a range plot (see *Range plots* later in this section). It does not calculate confidence intervals for you. You must provide two y values and one x value for each confidence interval. `rspike` would have plotted intervals without caps.

In figure 11.32, we entered the coordinates by using the `input` command. These coordinates were obtained from the original 140 observations by the `summarize` command, but they could be generated from the original dataset by using the `statsby` command; see section 17.1. The do-file `gph_fig11_32b.do` demonstrates how this can be done; it is accessible at this book's web site (http://www.stata-press.com/books/ishr2.html).

The dataset pkdata.dta is about drug concentration over time after ingestion.

```
. webuse pkdata
. summarize
```

Variable	Obs	Mean	Std. Dev.	Min	Max
id	208	10	5.972562	1	20
seq	208	1.5	.5012063	1	2
time	208	8.461538	9.637811	0	32
concA	208	4.698075	2.001099	0	8.382471
concB	208	5.159216	3.819005	0	14.37319

```
. sort id time
. list id time concA if id==1, separator(0)
```

	id	time	concA
1.	1	0	0
2.	1	.5	3.073403
3.	1	1	5.188444
4.	1	1.5	5.898577
5.	1	2	5.096378
6.	1	3	6.094085
7.	1	4	5.158772
8.	1	6	5.7065
9.	1	8	5.272467
10.	1	12	4.4576
11.	1	16	5.146423
12.	1	24	4.947427
13.	1	32	1.920421

Figure 11.33 shows the development for eight persons. This was done in the following do-file by creating a scatterplot with no markers and with lines connecting the points. The dataset must be in long form and sorted according to person and time. Use the connect(L) option; the connect(l) option would also connect the last point for one person with the first point for the next, and we do not want that.

```
──────────────── gph_fig11_33.do ────────────────
* gph_fig11_33.do

webuse pkdata.dta, clear
sort id time
set scheme lean1

twoway scatter concA time if id<10       ///
    ,                                    ///
  msymbol(none) connect(L)               ///
  plotregion(margin(b=0))                ///
  xsize(3) ysize(2.2) scale(1.4)
```

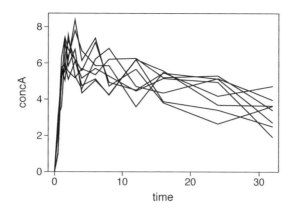

Figure 11.33. Lines illustrating individual development

With panel-data commands, you can obtain similar results; see [XT] **xtline**.

Range plots

Figure 11.32 included a range plot (`twoway rcap`). There are other range plots; see, e.g., [G] **graph twoway rarea**, [G] **graph twoway rbar**, [G] **graph twoway rcap**, [G] **graph twoway rline**, and [G] **graph twoway rspike**.

Dropped-line plots

A dropped-line plot is a plot with a line going from an observation point to a baseline; see [G] **graph twoway dropline**. Figure 11.34 aims to illustrate the observation time among 14 cancer patients who were monitored during a drug trial; the observation time may end with death or censoring.

(Continued on next page)

```
──────────────── gph_fig11_34.do ────────────────
* gph_fig11_34.do

sysuse cancer.dta      // Use the cancer.dta dataset accompanying Stata
keep if drug==2        // Study the 14 patients who received drug 2
sort studytime         // Sort by observation time
gen patient=_n         // and give numbers to patients

set scheme lean2

twoway                                                              ///
  (dropline studytime patient if died==1, horizontal msymbol(D))   ///
  (dropline studytime patient if died==0, horizontal msymbol(D)    ///
     mfcolor(white))                                                ///
  ,                                                                 ///
  plotregion(margin(l=0 b=0))                                       ///
  ytitle("Patient number")                                         ///
  yscale(range(0 14)) ylabel(1 5 10 14, nogrid)                    ///
  xtitle("Months after randomization")                             ///
  xlabel(0(6)30)                                                    ///
  legend(order(1 "Death" 2 "Censoring"))                           ///
  xsize(4.4) ysize(2.2) scale(1.4)
```

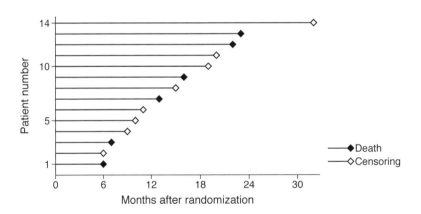

Figure 11.34. Dropped-line plot illustrating observation time in a drug trial

The baseline usually is the x or y axis or, rather, the line with x or $y = 0$, but you can define the baseline to be 5 with the base(5) option.

The marker for censorings is a diamond with white fill, not a hollow diamond, to avoid the dropped line's being visible within the marker.

Function plots

`twoway function` allows you to visualize mathematical functions; see [G] **graph twoway function**. Figure 11.35 is a normal distribution curve created using the `normalden()` function. For more information about mathematical functions, see [D] **functions**.

```
                              ———— gph_fig11_35.do ————
* gph_fig11_35.do

set scheme lean2

twoway                                          ///
  (function y=normalden(x), range(-3.5 3.5)     ///
    droplines(-1.96 -1 0 1 1.96))               ///
  ,                                             ///
  plotregion(margin(zero))                      ///
  yscale(off) ylabel(, nogrid)                  ///
  xlabel(-3 -1.96 -1 0 1 1.96 3, format(%4.2f)) ///
  xtitle("Standard deviations from mean")       ///
  xsize(3.3) ysize(2.2) scale(1.4)
```

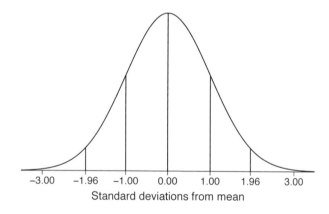

Figure 11.35. `twoway function` lets you plot, e.g., a normal curve

The `range()` option is mandatory; it defines the *x*-axis range. `droplines()` is an option to `function`, not a separate plot command. I set the plot-region margin to zero, to let the normal curve start at the baseline.

(Continued on next page)

Here are some other examples:

- An identity line to be overlaid on a scatterplot comparing two measurements (e.g., sbp1 and sbp2):

```
. twoway (scatter sbp2 sbp1)(function y=x, range(sbp1))
```

- A parabola:

```
. twoway (function y=x^2, range(-2 2))
```

Matrix graphs

Matrix scatterplots are useful for analysis but are rarely used for publication; see [G] **graph matrix**. They allow you to show the association between several variables in one graph.

```
─────────────────── gph_fig11_36.do ───────────────────
* gph_fig11_36.do

sysuse auto.dta
set scheme lean1

graph matrix price mpg weight length, xsize(5) ysize(4)
```

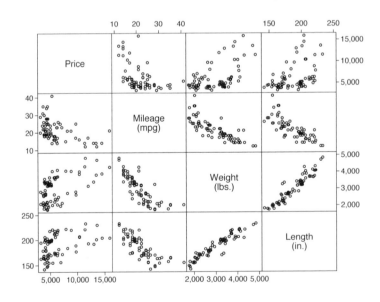

Figure 11.36. Matrix scatterplot

In figure 11.36, the upper-right cells are redundant rotated images of the lower-left cells. You can omit them by using the half option:

```
. graph matrix price mpg weight length, half
```

11.9 By-graphs and combined graphs

By-graphs

A by-graph is a graph split into two or more subgraphs; see [G] ***by_option***. The following do-file and figure 11.37 show a sample by-graph.

```
―――――――――――――――――― gph_fig11_37.do ――――――――――――
* gph_fig11_37.do

sysuse auto.dta
set scheme lean1

twoway (scatter mpg weight)        ///
   ,                               ///
   by(foreign, total note(""))     ///
   xsize(4.5) ysize(3.5)
```

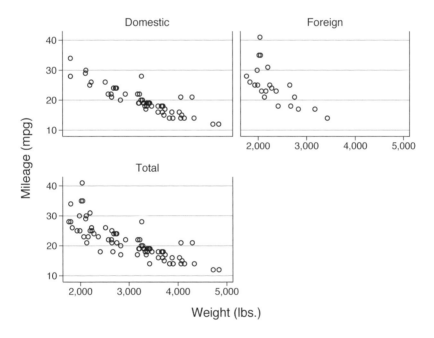

Figure 11.37. By-graph with the `total` option

The `total` suboption to the `by()` option displays the third graph with all observations. The `note("")` suboption removes a rather useless note ("Graphs by Car type"). You can let the graphs be stacked vertically by using the `cols()` suboption (`rows()` is used in a similar way):

```
. ..., by(foreign, cols(1))
```

Combining graphs

You can combine several graphs with the `graph combine` command. In figure 11.38, three graphs are created and then combined into one figure, as the following do-file shows.

```
──────────────── gph_fig11_38.do ────────────────
* gph_fig11_38.do

sysuse auto.dta
set scheme lean1

twoway (scatter mpg weight), name(scatter, replace)

histogram mpg, frequency horizontal name(h_mpg, replace)

histogram weight, frequency name(h_weight, replace)

graph combine scatter h_mpg h_weight, xsize(5) ysize(4)
```

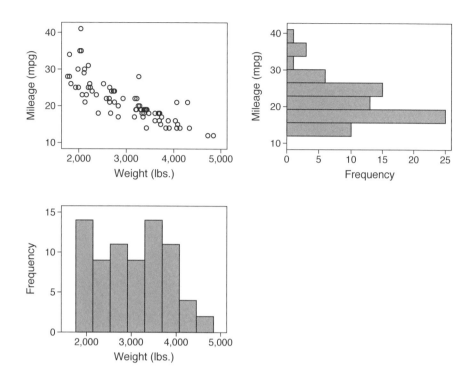

Figure 11.38. Combined graph

In figure 11.38, the individual graphs were stored as "memory graphs" by using the `name()` option. They are temporarily stored in computer memory without being written to disk. You can save them to disk with the `saving()` option:

. ..., `saving(scatter.gph, replace)`

You can combine them by typing

. `graph combine scatter.gph h_mpg.gph h_weight.gph`

Setting `xsize()` and `ysize()` for the individual graphs before combining has no effect on the final result. There are several advanced options for combining graphs; see [G] **graph combine**.

11.10 Using dialogs to generate commands

The menu and dialog system is very useful for producing graphs, especially to the less experienced user. Actually, it is more difficult to explain how to use the dialogs than to use them. Here I demonstrate how to develop the command creating figure 11.47. Take a look at the figure. It includes two plots, one with domestic and one with foreign cars, using data from the `auto.dta` dataset:

```
. sysuse auto.dta
```

Find the appropriate dialog by using the menus, clicking on

> Graphics ▷ Twoway graph (scatter, line, etc.)

or, when you know the command name, by typing, for example, the following command:

```
. db twoway
```

The general twoway dialog appears (see figure 11.39). Make sure the **Plots** tab is selected:

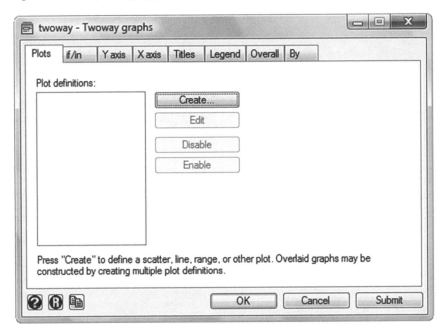

Figure 11.39. Twoway dialog

Click on the **Create...** button to get a dialog for the first plot. Select **Scatter**. From the drop-down lists, select mpg as the Y variable and weight as the X variable (see figure 11.40):

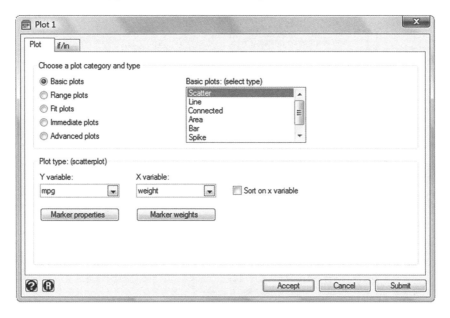

Figure 11.40. First plot dialog — **Plot** tab

(Continued on next page)

Next select the if/in tab. The first plot is for domestic cars (`foreign==0`). Type that in the expression field (see figure 11.41). Click on the **Accept** button.

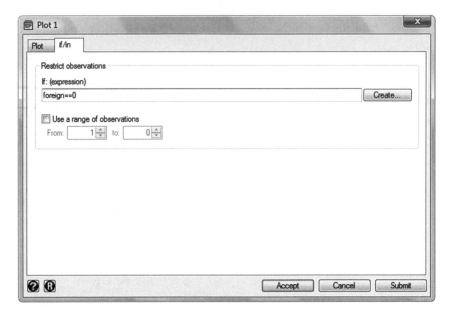

Figure 11.41. First plot dialog—if/in tab

Repeat the process for the second plot; it describes foreign cars (`foreign==1`).

After having defined the two plots, it is time to look at the entire graph. Use the Overall tab to determine the size of the graph (see figure 11.42):

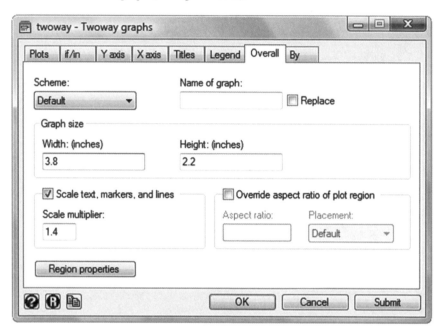

Figure 11.42. Twoway dialog — Overall tab

Now we want to see the result (see figure 11.43). Click on Submit rather than OK because Submit preserves the dialog and lets you make additional modifications, if desired:

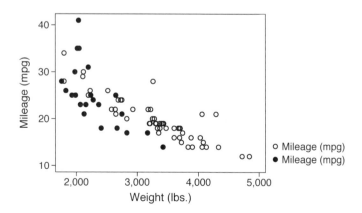

Figure 11.43. Graph defined by dialogs

Obviously, the legend is not informative and we want to modify it. Click on the Legend tab and enter the label specification (see figure 11.44):

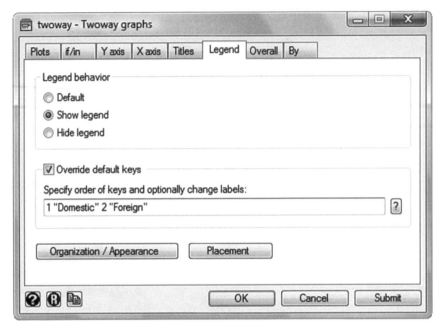

Figure 11.44. Twoway dialog — Legend tab

We also want a legend title. Click on the **Legend** dialog's **Organization/Appearance** button, select the **Titles** tab, and type the title (see figure 11.45):

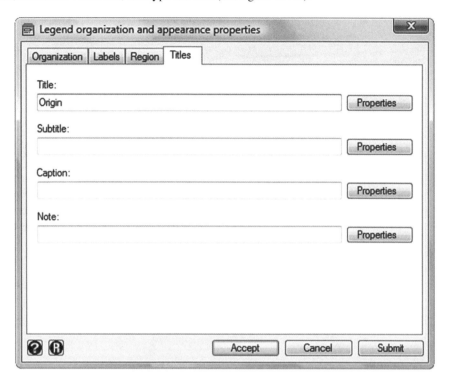

Figure 11.45. Legend organization and appearance properties

(Continued on next page)

Click on the **Submit** button to see the result. I found that the legend title font was too large; you can change this by clicking on the title field's **Properties** button. Here I entered the size specification *0.8 (see figure 11.46):

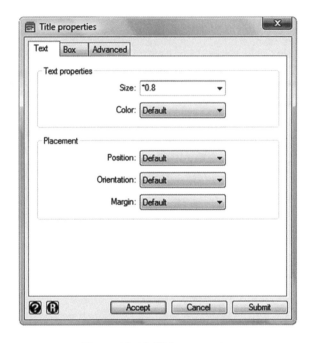

Figure 11.46. Title properties

Clicking on **Submit** displays the result (see figure 11.47).

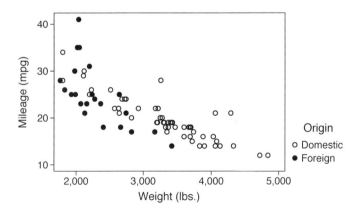

Figure 11.47. Graph defined by dialogs, with an improved legend

The dialogs generate commands, and the above sequence of actions displayed this command in the Results window:

```
. twoway (scatter mpg weight if foreign==0) (scatter mpg weight
> if foreign==1), legend(on order(1 "Domestic" 2 "Foreign")
> title(Origin, size(*0.8))) xsize(3.8) ysize(2.2) scale(1.4)
```

Once you are satisfied with the looks of a graph, save the commands that generated it as a do-file. You can do that from the Review window; see section 1.4. Edit the do-file to make it more legible, and then save it:

```
———————————————— gph_fig11_47.do ————————————————
* gph_fig11_47.do

sysuse auto.dta

twoway (scatter mpg weight if foreign==0) ///
(scatter mpg weight if foreign==1) ,      ///
legend(on order(1 "Domestic" 2 "Foreign") ///
title(Origin, size(*0.8)))                ///
xsize(3.8) ysize(2.2) scale(1.4)
```

11.11   The Graph Editor

So far, I have shown how to modify and fine-tune a graph's appearance by modifying the graph command creating it. This method has the advantage that each graph is unambiguously defined. You can reproduce it exactly, and you can make further well-defined modifications.

The Graph Editor lets you make modifications somewhat more intuitively. The modifications you make with the Graph Editor are not reflected in a modified command, but you can record your actions, and they can be replayed at a later time, maybe to modify an other graph.

The Graph Editor is used to modify existing graphs, not to create new graphs. You can use the Editor to move objects, modify objects, and insert new objects like textboxes, lines, and arrows. You must start with a graph in the Graph Window and then click on the Graph Editor button, ![icon]. See figure 11.48.

(Continued on next page)

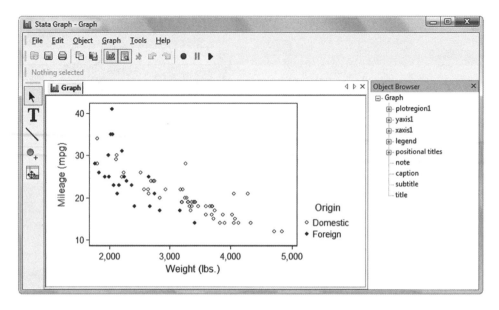

Figure 11.48. The Graph Editor

If you want to record your actions, click on the **Recording** button, 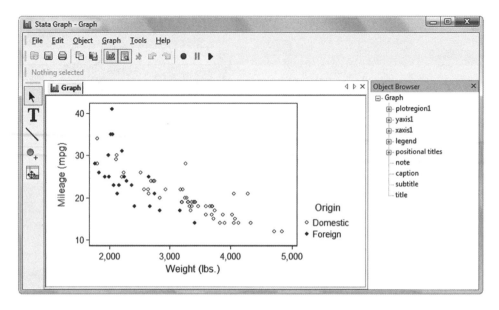, before doing anything else. I will tell more about the use of recordings at the end of this section.

The Object Browser to the right of the graph area gives an overview of the objects in the
graph. In the Object Browser, I selected title, and this opened a Contextual Toolbar above the
graph area. Here I entered a title for the graph (see figure 11.49) because the original graph had
no title. I could also have modified the title's font size and color. If you click on More... in
the Contextual Toolbar or right-click on an object, you get a dialog box where you can further
modify the object's properties.

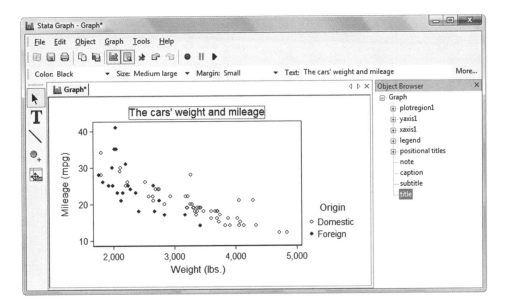

Figure 11.49. Graph with added title

To the left of the graph area you see five tool buttons. The Pointer Tool, ![pointer], is used to select and move objects. For example, you can select a title and drag it to another position while holding down the left mouse button. You can constrain the movements to vertical and horizontal direction by pressing the *Shift* key while dragging.

You cannot move objects related to data, e.g., markers in a scatterplot. This is different from packages like Microsoft Excel, which will alter the data if a point is moved on a graph. I find Stata's behavior strongly preferable.

With the Add Text Tool, **T**, you can add text to the graph by clicking anywhere in the graph area. Right-click on the text to get a dialog box if you want to modify the appearance of the text. Select the Pointer Tool and drag the textbox if you want to move it.

The Add Line Tool, ![line], lets you add lines and arrows. Click in the graph to establish the starting point, and drag to the ending point while holding down the left mouse button. Right-click on the line to modify it; one of the things you can do is add arrowheads. Select the Pointer Tool and drag the line if you want to move it. I added an arrow by using the Add Line Tool and a small textbox by using the Add Text Tool (see figure 11.50). These two elements are now displayed in the Object Browser.

(Continued on next page)

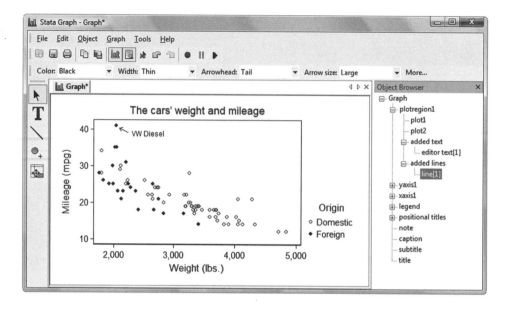

Figure 11.50. Graph with added line and text

With the Add Marker Tool, 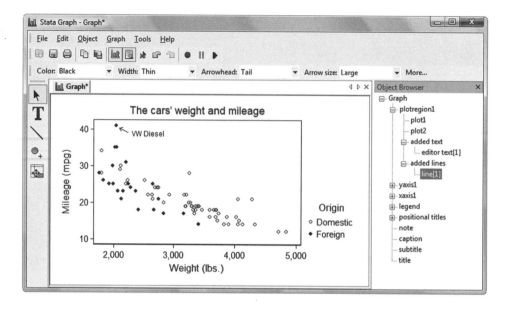 +, you can add a marker to the graph. Right-click on the marker if you want to modify it. Select the Pointer Tool and drag the marker if you want to move it. Dragging is only possible for markers added by the Graph Editor, not for markers related to data.

The last tool, the Grid Edit Tool, is not described here.

After modifications, you must save the modified graph. Click on the Save button, , or use File ▷ Save as...

If you recorded your actions, stop the recordings by clicking on the Recording button, , again. Read more in the following subsection.

This short introduction should help you get started using the Graph Editor. Find a more detailed tutorial by typing:

```
. help graph editor
```

It includes a section called *Tips, tricks, and quick edits*, which contains a number of good ideas.

Replaying recorded actions

When you stop recording by clicking on the Recording button, , you are asked if you want to save the recordings in a file. Such files have the extension .grec, and they are saved by default in the grec subfolder under your PERSONAL folder, typically in C:\ado\personal\grec, but you may choose to place it elsewhere.

You can inspect the file in the Do-file Editor, but do not expect to understand it, and respect the warning:

```
// Edit only if you know what you are doing
```

You can reuse the recordings in three ways:

- Open a graph in the Graph Editor, and then click on the Play button, ▶ .
- Include a play() option in the graph command, for example,

    ```
    . twoway scatter mpg weight, play(xyz.grec)
    ```
- When a graph is open, use the graph play command, for example,

    ```
    . graph play xyz.grec
    ```

11.12   Saving, displaying, and printing graphs

Saving a graph

You can save the current graph as a .gph file (for example, lifeexp.gph) by typing

```
. graph save lifeexp.gph [, asis replace]
```

The asis option saves a "frozen" graph, meaning that it is displayed as is, regardless of scheme settings. Without this option, you save a "live" graph: you can display it again, maybe using a different scheme or modifying its size, or you can edit it with the Graph Editor.

You can also include a saving() option within the graph command:

```
. ..., saving(lifeexp.gph, replace)
```

A saved graph can be displayed by typing

```
. graph use lifeexp.gph
```

Save a do-file for each graph

I strongly recommend that you save a do-file for each graph, with a name that tells what it does, e.g., gph_lifeexp.do. I recommend (Stata does not care) that you name all graph-defining do-files with a gph prefix, for easy identification. The do-file documents what you did; you can edit it to modify the graph, and you can modify it to create another graph. Remember to include the data or a use command reading the data used. This advice also applies when you have initially defined the graph command with a graph dialog.

Displaying and printing a graph

Redisplay the current graph by typing

```
. graph display [, scale(1.2) ysize(3) xsize(5) scheme(lean2)]
```

The `scale()` option is useful for increasing marker and text size, for example, for a slide show. `xsize()` and `ysize()` modify the size of the graph area (arguments in inches), and `scheme()` lets you display a graph under a different scheme — but that sometimes fails.

Copying and printing smooth colored or gray areas sometimes give poor results, and a coarser raster pattern may be needed. This is a printer issue, not a Stata issue, and in this respect modern printers are worse than older. If you encounter problems, you may experiment with selecting a coarser resolution, e.g., 300 dpi, rather than the now typical 600 or 1,200 dpi.

If you, in the future, do not want Stata's logo being printed on each graph, type

```
. graph set print logo off
```

Copying a graph to a document

To copy and paste a graph to another document, right-click in the Graph window, and select Copy Graph. Paste it to the document with Paste Special. In a Windows environment, the graph will be transferred as a metafile; there are two types, which you may select via the Graph Preferences menu:

> Edit ▷ Preferences ▷ Graph Preferences...

Select Enhanced Metafile (EMF) or Windows Metafile (WMF). The one that works best depends on your system and printer, so take a critical look at the results.

Submitting graphs to journals, etc.

The requirements of journals vary, but the best graph results are obtained by Encapsulated PostScript (`.eps`). The following command exports the current graph (here `fig3.eps`) as an `.eps` file:

```
. graph export fig3.eps, as(eps) replace
```

Windows metafiles (`.wmf`, `.emf`) give a reasonable quality, whereas formats such as Portable Network Graphics (`.png`) and TIFF (`.tif`) give poor results. For updated information on exporting graphs, see

```
. help graph export
```

12 Stratified analysis

Stratified analysis and standardization are related methods for controlling confounding due to an imbalance between the groups to be compared. The general principle is stratification by the potential confounder followed by calculation of a weighted average of the information. Standardization is described in section 14.6. Examples of other stratified analyses can be found in sections 12.1 and 12.2. Stratified analysis of incidence-rate data is described in section 14.1.

In this chapter, I also briefly mention the regression models corresponding to the stratified analysis commands. Regression analysis is demonstrated in more detail in chapter 13.

The commands in the `epitab` family perform various analyses of tabular data, including stratified analysis (Mantel–Haenszel). These commands are documented in [ST] **epitab**. The main `epitab` commands are shown in table 12.1.

Table 12.1. `epitab` commands

Command	Measure of association	See section	Immediate command (section 10.5)
`ir`	Incidence-rate ratio and difference	14.1	`iri`
`cs`	Cohort studies: Risk ratio and difference	12.1	`csi`
`cc`	Case–control studies: Odds ratio	12.2	`cci`
`tabodds`	Odds ratio: Multiple exposure levels	12.2	
`mhodds`	Odds ratio: Continuous exposure levels	12.2	
`mcc`	Odds ratio: matched case–control data	12.2	`mcci`

> Note: For most `epitab` commands, the unexposed and the noncases must be coded 0 to work correctly.

12.1 Cohort data without censorings

In cohort data without censorings, the absolute risk, relative risk, and risk difference can be estimated by using `cs` (cohort study).

The `ugdp.dta` dataset describes the results from a drug trial among diabetics (University Group Diabetes Program 1970). The exposure (exposed) is tolbutamide, and the outcome (case) is death within a defined time period. The dataset is in tabular form, with pop indicating the number of subjects in each cell.

```
. webuse ugdp.dta
. numlabel, add
. list, sepby(age)
```

	age	case	exposed	pop
1.	0. <55	0	0	115
2.	0. <55	0	1	98
3.	0. <55	1	0	5
4.	0. <55	1	1	8
5.	1. 55+	0	0	69
6.	1. 55+	0	1	76
7.	1. 55+	1	0	16
8.	1. 55+	1	1	22

Here is the result of a crude analysis, one not stratified or adjusted for anything. When analyzing a tabular dataset, you must specify the cell frequencies by using [fweight=*varname*] (see section 4.5):

```
. cs case exposed [fweight=pop]
```

	exposed Exposed	Unexposed	Total	
Cases	30	21	51	
Noncases	174	184	358	
Total	204	205	409	
Risk	.1470588	.102439	.1246944	
	Point estimate		[95% Conf. Interval]	
Risk difference	.0446198		-.0192936	.1085332
Risk ratio	1.435574		.8510221	2.421645
Attr. frac. ex.	.3034146		-.1750577	.5870576
Attr. frac. pop	.1784792			

chi2(1) =   1.87 Pr>chi2 = 0.1720

The crude analysis displays the risk difference (RD = 0.045; 95% CI: −0.019, 0.109) and the relative risk (RR = 1.44; 95% CI: 0.85, 2.42). The attributable risk among the exposed is 0.30. The interpretation is that, among the exposed, 30% of the cases would have been avoided in the absence of the exposure. In this study, the population attributable risk has no reasonable interpretation because the exposure prevalence is determined by the proportion (50%) allocated to treatment.

Using the information in the table, the immediate command `csi` gives the same result:

```
. csi 30 21 174 184
```

Now let's stratify by age:

```
. table case exposed [fweight=pop], by(age) row col
```

```
Age
category         exposed
and case       0      1   Total

0. <55
       0     115     98    213
       1       5      8     13

   Total     120    106    226

1. 55+
       0      69     76    145
       1      16     22     38

   Total      85     98    183
```

```
. cs case exposed [fweight=pop], by(age)
```

Age category	RR	[95% Conf. Interval]		M-H Weight
0. <55	1.811321	.6112044	5.367898	2.345133
1. 55+	1.192602	.6712664	2.11883	8.568306
Crude	1.435574	.8510221	2.421645	
M-H combined	1.325555	.797907	2.202132	

Test of homogeneity (M-H)   chi2(1) =   0.447 Pr>chi2 = 0.5037

The stratification gave a modest change in the RR estimate. The difference in RRs between the young and the old may be more important (question of interaction or effect modification). However, the test of homogeneity $(Pr = 0.50)$ leads us to accept a null hypothesis of a common relative risk.

It is commonplace to use logistic regression (see section 13.2) to analyze cohort data that have relative risk as the "natural" measure of association. Logistic regression, however, estimates the odds ratio, which only approximates the relative risk well under some circumstances. Binomial regression estimates relative risk directly (use `binreg` with the `rr` option). `nolog` reduces the amount of output:

(Continued on next page)

```
. binreg case exposed age [fweight=pop], rr nolog
Generalized linear models                    No. of obs       =       409
Optimization      : MQL Fisher scoring       Residual df      =       406
                    (IRLS EIM)               Scale parameter  =         1
Deviance          =  285.3425017             (1/df) Deviance  =   .702814
Pearson           =  405.3098098             (1/df) Pearson   =     .9983

Variance function: V(u) = u*(1-u)            [Bernoulli]
Link function    : g(u) = ln(u)              [Log]

                                             BIC              = -2156.226
```

		EIM				
case	Risk Ratio	Std. Err.	z	P>|z|	[95% Conf. Interval]	
exposed	1.310979	.3408281	1.04	0.298	.7875904	2.182182
age	3.535708	1.081063	4.13	0.000	1.941854	6.437781

The relative risk for exposure (RR = 1.31; 95% CI: 0.79, 2.18) is close to the result of the stratified analysis with cs.

binreg with the rd option estimates risk differences:

```
. binreg case exposed age [fweight=pop], rd nolog
Generalized linear models                    No. of obs       =       409
Optimization      : MQL Fisher scoring       Residual df      =       406
                    (IRLS EIM)               Scale parameter  =         1
Deviance          =  284.8924278             (1/df) Deviance  =  .7017055
Pearson           =  408.9955588             (1/df) Pearson   =  1.007378

Variance function: V(u) = u*(1-u)            [Bernoulli]
Link function    : g(u) = u                  [Identity]

                                             BIC              = -2156.676
```

		EIM				
case	Coef.	Std. Err.	z	P>|z|	[95% Conf. Interval]	
exposed	.0343372	.0278726	1.23	0.218	-.0202922	.0889666
age	.147714	.0337239	4.38	0.000	.0816164	.2138116
_cons	.041489	.0175319	2.37	0.018	.0071272	.0758508

Although it may be easier to communicate relative risks than odds ratios, analysis of binary outcomes is usually presented as odds ratios, which have nicer mathematical properties. For an instructive discussion, see Kirkwood and Sterne (2003).

12.2   Case–control data

cc: Dichotomous exposure

In a case–control study, the odds ratio can be estimated with cc (case–control). The unexposed and the noncases must be coded 0 for cc and cs to work correctly. We use the lbw1.dta dataset, studying the association between smoking and low birthweight.

In a case–control study, the exposure distribution among a group of cases is compared with the exposure distribution in the source population (the population that is the source of the cases). However, the source population is represented by a sample: the control subjects. From this design, the absolute disease risk cannot be estimated, but the relative risk can be approximated by using the odds-ratio estimate. To study the association between smoking and low birthweight, we first do a crude analysis without stratification:

```
. cd C:\docs\ishr2
c:\docs\ishr2

. use lbw1.dta
(Hosmer & Lemeshow data)

. cc low smoke
```

	Exposed	Unexposed	Total	Proportion Exposed
Cases	30	29	59	0.5085
Controls	44	86	130	0.3385
Total	74	115	189	0.3915

	Point estimate	[95% Conf. Interval]	
Odds ratio	2.021944	1.029092	3.965864 (exact)
Attr. frac. ex.	.5054264	.0282695	.7478481 (exact)
Attr. frac. pop	.2569965		

```
                   chi2(1) =    4.92  Pr>chi2 = 0.0265
```

The crude association is OR = 2.02 (95% CI: 1.03, 3.97). The attributable risk among the exposed is 0.51, meaning that, among the exposed, 51% of the cases would have been avoided in the absence of the exposure. To estimate the attributable risk in the population, the population exposure prevalence is estimated from the proportion exposed in the control group. In the absence of the exposure, 26% of all cases would have been avoided, provided that the association is causal.

Using the information in the table, we can see that the immediate command cci gives the same result:

```
. cci 30 29 44 86
```

The association between smoking and birthweight might be confounded by race. A direct way to examine this is by doing a stratified analysis. The by(race) option defines the stratification variable. Below are a three-way table of the data and a stratified analysis with cc.

(Continued on next page)

```
. table low smoke, by(race) row col stubwidth(15)
```

race and birthweight<2500g	smoked during pregnancy 0. No	1. Yes	Total
1. white			
0. No	40	33	73
1. Yes	4	19	23
Total	44	52	96
2. black			
0. No	11	4	15
1. Yes	5	6	11
Total	16	10	26
3. other			
0. No	35	7	42
1. Yes	20	5	25
Total	55	12	67

```
. cc low smoke, by(race)
```

race	OR	[95% Conf. Interval]		M-H Weight	
1. white	5.757576	1.657574	25.1388	1.375	(exact)
2. black	3.3	.4865385	23.45437	.7692308	(exact)
3. other	1.25	.273495	5.278229	2.089552	(exact)
Crude	2.021944	1.029092	3.965864		(exact)
M-H combined	3.086381	1.49074	6.389949		

```
Test of homogeneity (M-H)      chi2(2) =       3.03  Pr>chi2 = 0.2197
                    Test that combined OR = 1:
                            Mantel-Haenszel chi2(1) =         9.41
                                        Pr>chi2 =     0.0022
```

Without stratification, the odds ratio (crude OR) is 2.02 (95% CI: 1.03, 3.97), whereas the Mantel–Haenszel adjusted odds ratio is 3.09 (95% CI: 1.49, 6.39). The odds ratios for the three strata are rather different, but the confidence intervals are wide, and the test of homogeneity $(\text{Pr} = 0.22)$ does not reject the hypothesis that they represent a common odds ratio (question of interaction or effect modification).

You can stratify by one variable only, but the following egen command lets you generate a new variable (htrace) combining the categories of two variables (ht and race). The label option generates value labels for the new variable.

```
. egen htrace=group(ht race), label
. cc low smoke, by(htrace)
```

group(ht race)	OR	[95% Conf. Interval]		M-H Weight	
0. No 1. white	5.346774	1.505951	23.66822	1.362637	(exact)
0. No 2. black	3.125	.3992806	25.30971	.6956522	(exact)
0. No 3. other	1.428571	.3072007	6.120892	1.888889	(exact)
1. Yes 1. white	.	0	.	0	(exact)
1. Yes 2. black	.	0	.	0	(exact)
1. Yes 3. other	.	.	.	0	(exact)
Crude	2.021944	1.029092	3.965864		(exact)
M-H combined	3.265972	1.553342	6.866853		

```
Test of homogeneity (B-D)     chi2(5) =     2.87  Pr>chi2 = 0.7196
                       Test that combined OR = 1:
                               Mantel-Haenszel chi2(1) =      9.83
                                              Pr>chi2 =    0.0017
```

The example illustrates that there are limits to stratification: three strata (those with hypertension) become so thin that they contribute no information. In such cases, a regression model is preferable.

The regression model corresponding to stratified analysis of case–control data is logistic regression (see section 13.2), which also estimates odds ratios.

```
. xi: logistic low smoke ht i.race
i.race              _Irace_1-3        (naturally coded; _Irace_1 omitted)
```

```
Logistic regression                      Number of obs   =        189
                                         LR chi2(4)      =      18.32
                                         Prob > chi2     =     0.0011
Log likelihood = -108.17506              Pseudo R2       =     0.0781
```

low	Odds Ratio	Std. Err.	z	P>|z|	[95% Conf. Interval]	
smoke	3.094613	1.155266	3.03	0.002	1.488812	6.432395
ht	3.252896	2.028429	1.89	0.059	.9582548	11.04229
_Irace_2	2.803324	1.393426	2.07	0.038	1.058213	7.426313
_Irace_3	3.06541	1.240313	2.77	0.006	1.387008	6.774827

tabodds: Multiple exposure levels

To study the effect of multiple exposure levels in a case–control study, use tabodds; see [ST] **epitab**. The data are from the much-cited Ille-et-Vilaine study of risk factors for esophageal cancer (Breslow and Day 1993). The alcohol consumption (grams/day) is recorded in four levels. freq is the number of cases or controls in each exposure category, hence [fweight=freq] in the tabodds command. The or option displays odds ratios. Without it, tabodds displays absolute odds, which in a case–control study reflect design decisions more than anything else:

```
. webuse bdesop.dta, clear
. numlabel, add
. tabodds case alcohol [fweight=freq], or
```

alcohol	Odds Ratio	chi2	P>chi2	[95% Conf. Interval]	
1. 0-39	1.000000	.	.	.	.
2. 40-79	3.565271	32.70	0.0000	2.237981	5.679744
3. 80-119	7.802616	75.03	0.0000	4.497054	13.537932
4. 120+	27.225705	160.41	0.0000	12.507808	59.262107

```
Test of homogeneity (equal odds): chi2(3)  =   158.79
                                   Pr>chi2  =    0.0000
Score test for trend of odds:      chi2(1)  =   152.97
                                   Pr>chi2  =    0.0000
```

The tests of homogeneity and trend in tabodds refer to the dose–response association, whereas in most other commands, they refer to differences between strata (effect modification, interaction).

To adjust by stratification for another exposure, use the adjust() option:

```
. tabodds case alcohol [fweight=freq], adjust(tobacco)
Mantel-Haenszel odds ratios adjusted for tobacco
```

alcohol	Odds Ratio	chi2	P>chi2	[95% Conf. Interval]	
1. 0-39	1.000000	.	.	.	.
2. 40-79	3.261178	28.53	0.0000	2.059764	5.163349
3. 80-119	6.771638	62.54	0.0000	3.908113	11.733306
4. 120+	19.919526	123.93	0.0000	9.443830	42.015528

```
Score test for trend of odds: chi2(1)  =   135.04
                              Pr>chi2  =    0.0000
```

The corresponding logistic regression analysis follows:

```
. xi: logistic case i.alcohol i.tobacco [fweight=freq]
i.alcohol          _Ialcohol_1-4      (naturally coded; _Ialcohol_1 omitted)
i.tobacco          _Itobacco_1-4      (naturally coded; _Itobacco_1 omitted)
```

```
Logistic regression                         Number of obs  =        975
                                            LR chi2(6)     =     159.13
                                            Prob > chi2    =     0.0000
Log likelihood =     -415.18                Pseudo R2      =     0.1608
```

case	Odds Ratio	Std. Err.	z	P>|z|	[95% Conf. Interval]	
_Ialcohol_2	3.402691	.7976312	5.22	0.000	2.149269	5.387091
_Ialcohol_3	7.373851	1.949248	7.56	0.000	4.392206	12.37958
_Ialcohol_4	24.04584	7.872427	9.71	0.000	12.65794	45.67904
_Itobacco_2	1.471323	.3113935	1.82	0.068	.9717577	2.227706
_Itobacco_3	1.529773	.3919808	1.66	0.097	.9258051	2.527751
_Itobacco_4	2.685142	.7770595	3.41	0.001	1.522776	4.734765

The odds-ratio estimate for _Ialcohol_2 corresponds to tabodds' odds ratio for the category 40–79 g/day, with the first category (0–39 g/day) being the reference. The estimates are not identical because of different estimation principles, but the general pattern remains.

mhodds: Continuous exposure levels

mhodds performs simple and stratified analysis for case–control data where the exposure variable is on a continuous scale. The odds ratio is interpreted as the odds ratio per unit increase in the exposure.

Although the exposure (alcohol) is not recorded as a continuous variable in the esophagus cancer data but rather as four exposure levels (coded 1–4), we will use these data for comparison with tabodds:

```
. mhodds case alcohol [fweight=freq]

Score test for trend of odds with alcohol

(The Odds Ratio estimate is an approximation to the odds ratio
for a one unit increase in alcohol)
```

Odds Ratio	chi2(1)	P>chi2	[95% Conf. Interval]	
2.951639	152.97	0.0000	2.486415	3.503910

The interpretation is that when using group 1 (0–39 g/day) as the reference category, the odds ratio for group 2 is 2.95, for group 3 it is $2.95^2 = 8.70$, and for group 4 it is $2.95^3 = 25.67$. You could compare these results with those found by tabodds and conclude that the results from the two analyses are similar. The score test for trend in tabodds gave exactly the same chi-squared value; that is no accident, as it is the same analysis.

You can make a stratified analysis (the by() option) and see the odds ratios for the alcohol–cancer association in each stratum, and the Mantel–Haenszel weighted common estimate:

(Continued on next page)

```
. mhodds case alcohol [fweight=freq], by(tobacco)
```
Score test for trend of odds with alcohol
by tobacco

(The Odds Ratio estimate is an approximation to the odds ratio
for a one unit increase in alcohol)

tobacco	Odds Ratio	chi2(1)	P>chi2	[95% Conf. Interval]	
1. 0-9	3.906025	88.00	0.0000	2.93832	5.19244
2. 10-19	2.359218	28.11	0.0000	1.71781	3.24012
3. 20-29	2.168829	12.00	0.0005	1.39956	3.36093
4. 30+	2.323704	15.36	0.0001	1.52429	3.54237

Mantel-Haenszel estimate controlling for tobacco

Odds Ratio	chi2(1)	P>chi2	[95% Conf. Interval]	
2.802198	135.04	0.0000	2.355175	3.334069

Test of homogeneity of ORs (approx): chi2(3) =   8.43
                                     Pr>chi2 = 0.0379

The adjusted odds ratio does not differ much from the crude estimate. Finally, you can see the test of homogeneity of odds ratios across strata; $p = 0.04$ (and this time it really is a test of homogeneity). You can conclude that there is a significant interaction (or effect-measure modification): the level of tobacco use modifies the effect of alcohol when using the odds-ratio as the effect measure, and you should probably avoid reporting a single odds-ratio estimate. The finding that those with the lowest exposure to a competing risk factor have the highest *relative* risk (or odds ratio) is common: the denominator in the relative-risk calculation is small. Looking at absolute risks might be informative, but usually case–control designs do not allow that.

You might also stratify for tobacco by including it as a third variable in the varlist. The result is the same, but with this syntax the individual strata and the test of homogeneity are not displayed.

```
. mhodds case alcohol tobacco [fweight=freq]
```
Score test for trend of odds with alcohol
controlling for tobacco

(The Odds Ratio estimate is an approximation to the odds ratio
for a one unit increase in alcohol)

Odds Ratio	chi2(1)	P>chi2	[95% Conf. Interval]	
2.802198	135.04	0.0000	2.355175	3.334069

The corresponding logistic regression analysis is

```
. xi: logistic case alcohol i.tobacco [fweight=freq]
i.tobacco          _Itobacco_1-4        (naturally coded; _Itobacco_1 omitted)

Logistic regression                              Number of obs   =         975
                                                 LR chi2(4)      =      157.61
                                                 Prob > chi2     =      0.0000
Log likelihood =    -415.937                     Pseudo R2       =      0.1593
```

case	Odds Ratio	Std. Err.	z	P>|z|	[95% Conf. Interval]	
alcohol	2.751469	.2610628	10.67	0.000	2.284555	3.313811
_Itobacco_2	1.461981	.3092472	1.80	0.073	.9658066	2.213059
_Itobacco_3	1.572017	.401791	1.77	0.077	.9525744	2.594271
_Itobacco_4	2.711107	.7831288	3.45	0.001	1.539108	4.775559

The odds ratio for alcohol does not differ much from what we found with mhodds. But whereas mhodds with the by() option made the effect modification quite visible, we might easily miss it with a regression analysis.

mhodds is more flexible than cc; e.g., it allows more than one stratification variable. The confidence intervals differ a bit because of different estimation principles.

```
. use lbw1.dta, clear
(Hosmer & Lemeshow data)

. mhodds low smoke, by(ht race)
Maximum likelihood estimate of the odds ratio
Comparing smoke==1 vs. smoke==0
by ht race

note: only 5 of the 6 strata formed in this analysis contribute
      information about the effect of the explanatory variable
```

ht	race	Odds Ratio	chi2(1)	P>chi2	[95% Conf. Interval]	
0. No	1. white	5.346774	8.62	0.0033	1.52411	18.75719
0. No	2. black	3.125000	1.60	0.2056	0.48575	20.10425
0. No	3. other	1.428571	0.29	0.5889	0.38923	5.24326
1. Yes	1. white	.	0.67	0.4142	.	.
1. Yes	2. black	.	0.50	0.4795	.	.
1. Yes	3. other	.	.	.	.	.

Mantel-Haenszel estimate controlling for ht and race

Odds Ratio	chi2(1)	P>chi2	[95% Conf. Interval]	
3.265972	9.83	0.0017	1.491248	7.152783

```
Test of homogeneity of ORs (approx): chi2(4)   =     2.61
                                     Pr>chi2   =   0.6254
```

mcc: Analyzing matched case–control data

Matching in case–control studies may be used to attempt to control for confounding and to improve study efficiency. However, matched case–control studies require special treatment to obtain valid results: the matched sets (a case and its matched controls) must be kept together in the analysis, using a set identifier as a stratification variable.

The `lowbirth.dta` dataset is a modification of the `lbw.dta` dataset. We now have 56 case–control pairs matched on age (a 1:1 match) (Hosmer and Lemeshow 2000). The key variables are `pairid` (each case and the matching control constitute a set), `low` (1: cases, 0: controls), and `smoke` (1: smokers, 0: nonsmokers):

```
. webuse lowbirth.dta, clear
(Applied Logistic Regression, Hosmer & Lemeshow)

. keep pairid low smoke

. list in 1/6, sepby(pairid)
```

	pairid	low	smoke
1.	1	0	0
2.	1	1	1
3.	2	0	0
4.	2	1	0
5.	3	0	0
6.	3	1	0

This dataset is in long format, but the `mcc` command requires a wide format with the information on a case and its matching control in the same observation. We use `reshape` (see section 9.6) to convert the data to wide format:

```
. reshape wide smoke, i(pairid) j(low)
(note: j = 0 1)
```

Data	long	->	wide
Number of obs.	112	->	56
Number of variables	3	->	3
j variable (2 values)	low	->	(dropped)
xij variables:			
	smoke	->	smoke0 smoke1

```
. list in 1/3
```

	pairid	smoke0	smoke1
1.	1	0	1
2.	2	0	0
3.	3	0	0

Each observation now constitutes a set, with `smoke0` containing information on exposure of the control and `smoke1` containing the exposure of the case. To perform the analysis, type

```
. mcc smoke1 smoke0
```

	Controls		
Cases	Exposed	Unexposed	Total
Exposed	8	22	30
Unexposed	8	18	26
Total	16	40	56

```
McNemar's chi2(1) =       6.53    Prob > chi2 = 0.0106
Exact McNemar significance probability      = 0.0161
```

Proportion with factor

Cases	.5357143	
Controls	.2857143	[95% Conf. Interval]

difference	.25	.0519726	.4480274	
ratio	1.875	1.148685	3.060565	
rel. diff.	.35	.1336258	.5663742	
odds ratio	2.75	1.179154	7.143667	(exact)

mcc performs McNemar's test for matched pairs and displays several estimates of which the odds ratio is the most interesting (OR = 2.75; 95% CI: 1.18, 7.14).

Using the information in the table, we can see that the immediate command mcci gives the same result:

```
. mcci 8 22 8 18
```

mcc simply performed an analysis stratifying by pairid. In the output above, we see 22 + 8 informative pairs, while the 8 + 18 pairs with the same exposure for cases and controls provide no information. The odds-ratio estimate is 22/8 = 2.75. We can obtain almost the same estimate with cc without a reshape; the confidence intervals differ somewhat. mcc's exact confidence interval is the most accurate.

```
. webuse lowbirth.dta
(Applied Logistic Regression, Hosmer & Lemeshow)
. cc low smoke, by(pairid)
```

Case-control pai	OR	[95% Conf. Interval]		M-H Weight	
1	.	0	.	0	(exact)
2	.	.	.	0	(exact)
(output omitted)					
55	.	0	.	0	(exact)
56	.	0	.	0	(exact)
Crude	2.884615	1.232782	6.820096		(exact)
M-H combined	2.75	1.224347	6.176763		

```
Test of homogeneity (Tarone)   chi2(55) =    50.00  Pr>chi2 = 0.6656

                 Test that combined OR = 1:
                         Mantel-Haenszel chi2(1) =      6.53
                                        Pr>chi2 =    0.0106
```

cc produced quite a long and not very informative table with 56 strata. You can obtain the same information without the table — and get some additional information — by using mhodds:

```
. mhodds low smoke pairid
```

Mantel-Haenszel estimate of the odds ratio
Comparing smoke==1 vs. smoke==0, controlling for pairid

note: only 30 of the 56 strata formed in this analysis contribute
      information about the effect of the explanatory variable

Odds Ratio	chi2(1)	P>chi2	[95% Conf. Interval]	
2.750000	6.53	0.0106	1.224347	6.176763

The appropriate regression model for matched case–control data is conditional logistic regression. Whereas we analyzed 1:1 matched data above, clogit analyzes any matching ratio, including varying number of controls, and it allows controlling for more confounders; see section 13.4.

```
. clogit low smoke, group(pairid) or nolog
```

Conditional (fixed-effects) logistic regression

			Number of obs	=	112
			LR chi2(1)	=	6.79
			Prob > chi2	=	0.0091
Log likelihood = -35.419282			Pseudo R2	=	0.0875

low	Odds Ratio	Std. Err.	z	P>|z|	[95% Conf. Interval]	
smoke	2.75	1.135369	2.45	0.014	1.224347	6.176763

13 Regression analysis

This chapter describes the fundamentals of linear regression and logistic regression. There are, however, many other regression models available in Stata. Chapter 14 discusses Poisson regression and Cox regression, and the general principles apply to them, too.

Performing regression analysis with Stata is easy. Defining regression models that make sense and interpreting the results are more complex. Especially consider the following:

- If you study a causal hypothesis, then make sure that your model is meaningful. Do not include independent variables that may represent steps in the causal pathway because they may create more confounding than they prevent. Automatic selection procedures are available in Stata (see [R] **stepwise**), but they may seduce the user into not thinking. I will, therefore, not describe them.

- If your hypothesis is noncausal and you look only for predictors, then logical requirements are more relaxed, but at least the time relations should be meaningful.

- Take care with closely associated independent variables, such as education and social class. Including both may obscure more information than it illuminates.

Kirkwood and Sterne (2003) give good advice on several general issues in regression modeling.

13.1 Linear regression

A linear regression expresses the dependency of one variable (the response, outcome, or dependent variable) on one or more other variables (predictors, regressors, or independent variables). For extensive documentation, see [R] **regress**.

We use the `auto.dta` dataset. With `mpg` (mileage) as the dependent variable and `weight` as a predictor, the `regress` command gives the following output:

```
. sysuse auto.dta
(1978 Automobile Data)

. regress mpg weight

      Source |       SS       df       MS              Number of obs =      74
-------------+------------------------------           F(  1,    72) =  134.62
       Model |  1591.9902        1   1591.9902          Prob > F      =  0.0000
    Residual |  851.469256      72  11.8259619          R-squared     =  0.6515
-------------+------------------------------           Adj R-squared =  0.6467
       Total |  2443.45946      73  33.4720474          Root MSE      =  3.4389

------------------------------------------------------------------------------
         mpg |      Coef.   Std. Err.      t    P>|t|     [95% Conf. Interval]
-------------+----------------------------------------------------------------
      weight |  -.0060087   .0005179   -11.60   0.000    -.0070411   -.0049763
       _cons |   39.44028   1.614003    24.44   0.000     36.22283    42.65774
------------------------------------------------------------------------------
```

The last part of the output with the regression coefficients is the most important. It can be translated to

$$\text{Predicted mpg (miles/gallon)} = 39.44 - 0.006 \times \texttt{weight}$$

A difference in weight of 1,000 lb. corresponds to a predicted difference in mileage of -6 miles per gallon. The 95% confidence interval is $(-7, -5)$ miles per gallon. The result is highly significant ($t = -11.6$; $\Pr < 0.001$). `_cons` is the constant or intercept, i.e., the predicted outcome when all predictors are 0. Here it is the predicted mileage (39.4 miles per gallon) for a car with a weight of 0 lb. Extrapolations outside the observed ranges of the predictors can lead to nonsense, but the intercept informs you about the general level of the outcome.

The R-squared statistic (R^2) of 0.65 is the *coefficient of determination* and is interpreted as the proportion of the variation in mileage that is "explained" by the cars' weights. In figure 13.1, a scatterplot with a regression line illustrates the association. Here we show the minimum graph command, but you can find a do-file with the full command (`gph_fig13_1.do`) at this book's web site:

```
. twoway (scatter mpg weight) (lfit mpg weight)
```

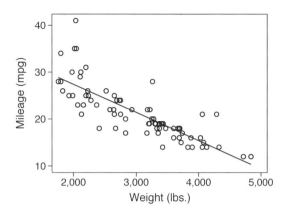

Figure 13.1. Scatterplot with a regression line

Regression diagnostics

The main requirements for a linear regression analysis to be valid are as follows:

- The association should be linear.

- The residuals (observed–predicted mpg) should be normally distributed.

- The variation of the residuals should be independent of the level of mpg (homoskedasticity).

You can read more in [R] **regress postestimation**. For more about postestimation commands in general, see [U] **20 Estimation and postestimation commands**.

Looking at the scatterplot in figure 13.1, we can see that the association is obvious, but a straight line may not be the best description. You can amend the residuals to the dataset by using the predict command just after the regression analysis, and you can examine the distribution in a histogram. predict (see [R] **predict**) is a postestimation command. From the regression coefficients, it creates a new variable: the predicted mpg for each observation. Use e(sample) to make sure that the prediction applies only to the observations included in the regression analysis (see figure 13.2):

(Continued on next page)

```
. predict pmpg if e(sample)
. label variable pmpg "Predicted mpg"
. generate rmpg = mpg - pmpg
. label variable rmpg "Residuals"
. histogram rmpg, frequency normal
```

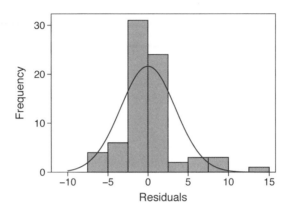

Figure 13.2. Histogram of residuals with normal curve overlaid

You could also obtain the residual directly with the following command:

```
. predict rmpg if e(sample), residual
```

The residual distribution in figure 13.2 does not seem to be normal. This supposition can be tested formally with the `swilk` command:

```
. swilk rmpg
```

	Shapiro-Wilk W test for normal data				
Variable	Obs	W	V	z	Prob>z
rmpg	74	0.89593	6.702	4.150	0.00002

The Shapiro–Wilk test leads us to reject the hypothesis that the residuals are from a normal distribution. However, with large datasets (this is not one), even unimportant departures from normality become significant, and visual inspection is the most important tool.

The requirement that the residual variation is constant across the predicted levels (homoskedasticity) can be examined by `rvfplot` (residual versus fitted; see figure 13.3). This command also should be issued after a regression analysis.

```
. rvfplot, yline(0)
```

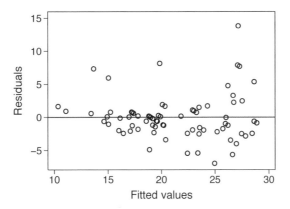

Figure 13.3. Residual-versus-fitted plot

The residual variation seems to increase with increasing predicted values of mpg, and the requirement of homoskedasticity is not fulfilled.

In conclusion, this was a case where the requirements for linear regression were not fulfilled, and, although we do not doubt that there is a strong association between the cars' weight and mileage, the linear regression model is probably not the best description. One possible solution is a transformation of the dependent variable. In section 10.4, the output from gladder led to the suggestion to make an inverse transformation of mpg; I chose to express it as gallons per 100 miles:

```
. generate gp100m = 100/mpg
. label variable gp100m "Gallons per 100 miles"
```

Now we could run a regression with gp100m as the dependent variable and look at the results. We could make a scatterplot like figure 13.1 and diagnostic plots like figures 13.2 and 13.3, and evaluate the results. Then we could compare the R^2 values from the two analyses.

Cox (2004) surveys a whole family of regression diagnostic graphs; you can find it by typing

```
. findit modeldiag
```

(Continued on next page)

Regression analysis with several independent variables

We will now turn to the `lbw1.dta` dataset on predictors of low birthweight. `describe` tells us about the dataset:

```
. cd C:\docs\ishr2
c:\docs\ishr2

. use lbw1.dta, clear
(Hosmer & Lemeshow data)

. describe

Contains data from C:\docs\ishr2\lbw1.dta
  obs:           189                          Hosmer & Lemeshow data
 vars:            11                          2 Apr 2005 21:10
 size:         3,402 (99.9% of memory free)

              storage  display    value
variable name   type   format     label     variable label

id              int    %8.0g                 identification code
low             byte   %8.0g      yesno      birthweight<2500g
age             byte   %8.0g                 age of mother
lwt             int    %8.0g                 weight at last menstrual period
race            byte   %8.0g      race       race
smoke           byte   %8.0g      yesno      smoked during pregnancy
ptl             byte   %8.0g                 premature labor history (count)
ht              byte   %8.0g      yesno      has history of hypertension
ui              byte   %8.0g      yesno      presence, uterine irritability
ftv             byte   %8.0g                 number of visits to physician
                                               during 1st trimester
bwt             int    %8.0g                 birthweight (grams)

Sorted by:
```

We hypothesize that maternal age (`age`), prepregnancy weight (`lwt`), and smoking (`smoke`) influence birthweight. Actually, smoking is the factor of interest, but smoking may be associated with maternal age and weight; without controlling for these factors, we might misinterpret the causal effect of smoking (a confounding problem). `age` and `lwt` are continuous variables, but `smoke` is dichotomous, and we must know how it is coded to interpret the results. Fortunately, we used `numlabel` to add codes to the value labels:

```
. tab1 smoke

-> tabulation of smoke

    smoked
    during
 pregnancy |      Freq.     Percent        Cum.

     0. No |        115       60.85       60.85
    1. Yes |         74       39.15      100.00

     Total |        189      100.00
```

```
. regress bwt age lwt smoke
```

Source	SS	df	MS
Model	7000336.31	3	2333445.44
Residual	92914962.3	185	502243.039
Total	99915298.6	188	531464.354

```
Number of obs =     189
F(  3,    185) =    4.65
Prob > F       =  0.0037
R-squared      =  0.0701
Adj R-squared =  0.0550
Root MSE       =  708.69
```

bwt	Coef.	Std. Err.	t	P>|t|	[95% Conf. Interval]
age	7.040796	9.923378	0.71	0.479	-12.53674 26.61833
lwt	4.020133	1.719721	2.34	0.020	.6273465 7.412919
smoke	-268.146	105.7908	-2.53	0.012	-476.8575 -59.43464
_cons	2363.765	300.6933	7.86	0.000	1770.537 2956.994

From the small $R^2 = 0.07$, we can see that these predictors explain only a small amount of the variation in birthweight. The association with age is insignificant, but there is a tendency toward increased birthweight with increasing maternal age (7 g per year). There is a significant association with the mother's prepregnancy weight (lwt) of 4 g per lb. The coefficient for smoke is -268 g (95% CI: -477, -59), meaning that, when controlling for maternal age and prepregnancy weight, smokers had babies that were on average 268 g lighter than those of nonsmokers.

With three independent variables, the relationship cannot be displayed graphically, but you can still calculate the residuals (predict) and use rvfplot to examine them.

Just after issuing the regression command, you can estimate the expected birthweight for, e.g., a newborn whose mother is 30 years old and had a prepregnancy weight of 120 lb.; see [R] **adjust**.

```
. adjust age=30 lwt=120, by(smoke) se ci
```

```
Dependent variable: bwt     Command: regress
Covariates set to value: age = 30, lwt = 120
```

smoked during pregnancy	xb	stdp	lb	ub
0. No	3057.41	(97.0107)	[2866.02	3248.79]
1. Yes	2789.26	(110.599)	[2571.06	3007.46]

```
Key:  xb        =  Linear Prediction
      stdp      =  Standard Error
      [lb , ub] =  [95% Confidence Interval]
```

The by(smoke) option shows the estimates for smokers and nonsmokers. To get a confidence interval, specify the ci option. If we had not specified values for age and lwt, they would be set to their mean values.

lincom can be used for similar purposes (see [R] **lincom**):

```
. lincom 30*age + 120*lwt + smoke + _cons

 ( 1)   30 age + 120 lwt + smoke + _cons = 0
```

bwt	Coef.	Std. Err.	t	P>|t|	[95% Conf. Interval]
(1)	2789.259	110.5992	25.22	0.000	2571.061 3007.457

The results from adjust and lincom depend on the preceding regression command. Here

```
. lincom 30*age + _cons
```

would be the same as

```
. lincom 30*age + 0*lwt + 0*smoke + _cons
```

so we get the predicted birthweight for 30-year-old nonsmoking mothers with a prepregnancy weight of 0!

Working with categorical predictors: The xi: prefix

Let's say we wish to include race in the list of predictors. The purpose can be to control for confounding by race when we are estimating the independent effect of smoking, or we may be interested in the effect of race itself on birthweight. The coding of race is

```
. tab1 race

-> tabulation of race
```

race	Freq.	Percent	Cum.
1. white	96	50.79	50.79
2. black	26	13.76	64.55
3. other	67	35.45	100.00
Total	189	100.00	

race is on a nominal scale. The codes themselves (1, 2, 3) are just codes, and there is no point in using them as values in any analysis. We want to contrast the birthweight among blacks and among others with that of white mothers. To do this, we need to construct dichotomous dummy or indicator variables. One way to do this is to let tab1 generate them. quietly suppresses the display of the table, and generate() creates a new dichotomous variable for each value of race. For the groups command, see section 10.3.

```
. quietly tab1 race, generate(race)

. groups race*
```

race	race1	race2	race3	Freq.	Percent
1. white	1	0	0	96	50.79
2. black	0	1	0	26	13.76
3. other	0	0	1	67	35.45

Now we can run the regression with the new dummy variables (race? means all variables starting with race and having exactly one more character):

```
. regress bwt smoke race?
```

Source	SS	df	MS		
Model	12346897.6	3	4115632.54		
Residual	87568400.9	185	473342.708		
Total	99915298.6	188	531464.354		

Number of obs = 189
F(3, 185) = 8.69
Prob > F = 0.0000
R-squared = 0.1236
Adj R-squared = 0.1094
Root MSE = 688

bwt	Coef.	Std. Err.	t	P>|t|	[95% Conf. Interval]	
smoke	-428.0254	109.0033	-3.93	0.000	-643.0746	-212.9761
race1	450.54	153.066	2.94	0.004	148.5607	752.5194
race2	(dropped)					
race3	-3.641269	160.537	-0.02	0.982	-320.3599	313.0773
_cons	2884.317	141.291	20.41	0.000	2605.569	3163.066

Stata dropped race2 from the analysis because it contributed no information beyond race1 and race3. The information in a variable with three categories can be expressed with two dummy variables. The effect was that race2 (blacks) became the reference group with which the birthweight of whites and others were compared. However, we want the whites to be the reference group—one good reason is that it is the largest group—so we omit this variable (race1) from the command.

```
. regress bwt smoke race2 race3
```

Source	SS	df	MS		
Model	12346897.6	3	4115632.54		
Residual	87568400.9	185	473342.708		
Total	99915298.6	188	531464.354		

Number of obs = 189
F(3, 185) = 8.69
Prob > F = 0.0000
R-squared = 0.1236
Adj R-squared = 0.1094
Root MSE = 688

bwt	Coef.	Std. Err.	t	P>|t|	[95% Conf. Interval]	
smoke	-428.0254	109.0033	-3.93	0.000	-643.0746	-212.9761
race2	-450.54	153.066	-2.94	0.004	-752.5194	-148.5607
race3	-454.1813	116.436	-3.90	0.000	-683.8944	-224.4683
_cons	3334.858	91.74301	36.35	0.000	3153.86	3515.855

The average birthweight among blacks (race2) was 451 g lower than among whites, and the birthweight among others (race3) was 454 g lower than among whites, when controlling for maternal smoking.

Stata has an elegant way to construct the dummy variables: by using the xi: prefix (see [R] **xi**):

```
. xi: regress bwt i.smoke i.race
i.smoke            _Ismoke_0-1       (naturally coded; _Ismoke_0 omitted)
i.race             _Irace_1-3        (naturally coded; _Irace_1 omitted)
```

Source	SS	df	MS
Model	12346897.6	3	4115632.54
Residual	87568400.9	185	473342.708
Total	99915298.6	188	531464.354

Number of obs =	189
F(3, 185) =	8.69
Prob > F =	0.0000
R-squared =	0.1236
Adj R-squared =	0.1094
Root MSE =	688

bwt	Coef.	Std. Err.	t	P>|t|	[95% Conf. Interval]	
_Ismoke_1	-428.0254	109.0033	-3.93	0.000	-643.0746	-212.9761
_Irace_2	-450.54	153.066	-2.94	0.004	-752.5194	-148.5607
_Irace_3	-454.1813	116.436	-3.90	0.000	-683.8944	-224.4683
_cons	3334.858	91.74301	36.35	0.000	3153.86	3515.855

This result is identical to that of the preceding analysis. xi: created three new dichotomous variables (coded 0/1): _Ismoke_1, _Irace_2, and _Irace_3. See the output from describe:

```
. describe
```
(output omitted)

variable name	storage type	display format	value label	variable label
id	int	%8.0g		identification code
(output omitted)				
_Ismoke_1	byte	%8.0g		smoke==1
_Irace_2	byte	%8.0g		race==2
_Irace_3	byte	%8.0g		race==3

```
Sorted by:
    Note:  dataset has changed since last saved
```

By default, the first (lowest) category will be omitted in the construction of dummy variables; here it means that nonsmokers (smoke = 0) and whites (race = 1) become the reference groups. If you wanted blacks (race = 2) to be the reference group, you could do that by assigning a "characteristic" to race (see [R] **xi**):

```
. char race[omit] 2
```

If you save the dataset, the dummy variables and characteristics are saved with it.

In the above regression, you see separate significance tests for _Irace2 (blacks versus whites) and _Irace3 (others versus whites). You might, however, want to test the overall difference between races. To do that, use `test` and `testparm` (see [R] **test**). Like `lincom`, you must run the command just after the estimation command. Here we find a significant overall difference in birthweight between races:

```
. quietly xi: regress bwt i.smoke i.race
. testparm _Irace*
 ( 1)  _Irace_2 = 0
 ( 2)  _Irace_3 = 0
       F(  2,   185) =    9.24
            Prob > F =    0.0001
```

Interactions in regression analysis

The effect of smoking on birthweight might be different among whites, blacks, and others. This phenomenon is called *interaction* or *effect modification*, and it can be studied by comparing the observed and predicted values of the dependent variable after running a regression analysis (the analysis shown above):

```
. quietly xi: regress bwt i.smoke i.race
. predict pbwt if e(sample)
(option xb assumed; fitted values)
. generate resid = bwt - pbwt
. table smoke, by(race) c(mean bwt mean pbwt mean resid) format(%8.0f)
> stubwidth(18)
```

race and smoked during pregnancy	mean(bwt)	mean(pbwt)	mean(resid)
1. white			
0. No	3429	3335	94
1. Yes	2827	2907	-79
2. black			
0. No	2854	2884	-30
1. Yes	2504	2456	48
3. other			
0. No	2814	2881	-66
1. Yes	2757	2453	305

For the observed values (`bwt`), you see a large difference between smoking and nonsmoking white women (602 g), whereas the difference is small (57 g) for women of "other" race. For the predicted values (`pbwt`), you see the same difference for all races (428 g). The regression model used assumes the same effect across races, and the discrepancies between observed and predicted values indicate that our model is too simple. There seems to be interaction between race and the effect of smoking (effect modification).

The `xi:` prefix also facilitates analyzing models with interactions:

```
. use lbw1, clear
(Hosmer & Lemeshow data)
. xi: regress bwt i.smoke*i.race
i.smoke           _Ismoke_0-1      (naturally coded; _Ismoke_0 omitted)
i.race            _Irace_1-3       (naturally coded; _Irace_1 omitted)
i.smoke*i.race    _IsmoXrac_#_#    (coded as above)
```

Source	SS	df	MS
Model	14455540.4	5	2891108.08
Residual	85459758.2	183	466993.214
Total	99915298.6	188	531464.354

```
Number of obs =      189
F(  5,    183) =     6.19
Prob > F       =   0.0000
R-squared      =   0.1447
Adj R-squared  =   0.1213
Root MSE       =   683.37
```

bwt	Coef.	Std. Err.	t	P>|t|	[95% Conf. Interval]	
_Ismoke_1	-601.3654	139.979	-4.30	0.000	-877.5456	-325.1851
_Irace_2	-574.25	199.5008	-2.88	0.004	-967.8674	-180.6326
_Irace_3	-614.5136	138.2182	-4.45	0.000	-887.2198	-341.8075
IsmoXrac~2	250.8654	308.9992	0.81	0.418	-358.7938	860.5245
IsmoXrac~3	544.2957	258.8455	2.10	0.037	33.59038	1055.001
_cons	3428.75	103.0218	33.28	0.000	3225.487	3632.013

The product `i.smoke*i.race` creates the main-effect dummy variables, as before, and two product (interaction) variables. The following table shows the values of the dummy and interaction variables for all combinations of the primary variables `smoke` and `race`. `groups` is an unofficial command; see section 10.3 for information on how to obtain it. `show(freq)` displays frequencies, and `abbrev(20)` prevents abbreviation of long variable names:

```
. groups smoke race _I*, sepby(smoke) show(freq) abbrev(20) nolabel
```

smoke	race	_Ismoke_1	_Irace_2	_Irace_3	_IsmoXrac_1_2	_IsmoXrac_1_3	Freq.
0	1	0	0	0	0	0	44
0	2	0	1	0	0	0	16
0	3	0	0	1	0	0	55
1	1	1	0	0	0	0	52
1	2	1	1	0	1	0	10
1	3	1	0	1	0	1	12

The significant interaction term `_IsmoXrac_1_3` expresses that the effect of smoking on birthweight was significantly different between whites and others; there is effect modification. Now a table of observed and predicted means shows no difference. The regression model is "saturated", that is, it includes all possible interaction terms between `smoke` and `race`:

```
. quietly xi: regress bwt i.smoke*i.race
. predict pbwt if e(sample)
(option xb assumed; fitted values)
. generate resid = bwt - pbwt
. table smoke, by(race) c(mean bwt mean pbwt mean resid) format(%8.0f)
> stubwidth(18)
```

race and smoked during pregnancy	mean(bwt)	mean(pbwt)	mean(resid)
1. white			
0. No	3429	3429	0
1. Yes	2827	2827	0
2. black			
0. No	2854	2854	0
1. Yes	2504	2504	0
3. other			
0. No	2814	2814	0
1. Yes	2757	2757	-0

The "perfect" fit does not rule out the importance of other factors not included in the model, and most of the variation in birthweight is not explained by the predictors. The adjusted R^2 (the coefficient of determination) is only 0.12, and the residual plot, figure 13.4, shows a lot of variation around the fitted (or predicted) values. The strange pattern is due to the simple fact that there are only six combinations of the predictors:

```
. rvfplot, yline(0)
```

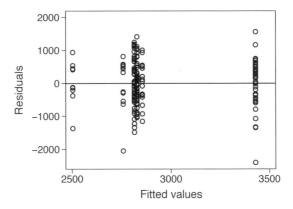

Figure 13.4. Residual-versus-fitted plot

Nested regression

When working with regression models, a frequent question is to what extent a more complex model adds information compared to a less complex model. In the preceding examples, we analyzed the effect of the mother's race and smoking habits on birthweight, and we examined whether an interaction term between smoking and race added to the prediction of birthweight. In a nested regression, we can build increasingly complex models and compare them.

The `nestreg` prefix command facilitates the analysis. In the following example, we examine the effect of race (block 1), next adding smoking to the model (block 2), and finally including interaction terms (block 3). The `quietly` option suppresses the output from the three regression analyses, but the final table gives an overview of the added information with increasingly complex models. I would not put too much weight on the p-values, but I would still conclude that the interaction between smoking and race is worth reporting.

```
. xi: nestreg, quietly: regress bwt (i.race) (i.smoke) (i.smoke*i.race)
i.race            _Irace_1-3          (naturally coded; _Irace_1 omitted)
i.smoke           _Ismoke_0-1         (naturally coded; _Ismoke_0 omitted)
i.smoke*i.race    _IsmoXrac_#_#       (coded as above)
note: _Ismoke_1 dropped because of collinearity
note: _Irace_2 dropped because of collinearity
note: _Irace_3 dropped because of collinearity

Block  1: _Irace_2 _Irace_3
Block  2: _Ismoke_1
Block  3: _IsmoXrac_1_2 _IsmoXrac_1_3
```

Block	F	Block df	Residual df	Pr > F	R2	Change in R2
1	4.95	2	186	0.0081	0.0505	
2	15.42	1	185	0.0001	0.1236	0.0730
3	2.26	2	183	0.1075	0.1447	0.0211

Note that the results depend strongly on the sequence of predictors included. That sequence is a prior decision. In the example, race is a stable property while smoking is a potentially modifiable behavior, so the race–smoking sequence seems reasonable. Inclusion of the more complex interaction term should be the last step, of course.

`nestreg` works with many regression commands, including `logistic`, `poisson`, and `stcox`, all demonstrated later in this book. Read more in [R] **nestreg**.

13.2   Logistic regression

In a logistic regression analysis, the outcome is binary. The probability (p) is expressed as *odds*, i.e., $p/(1-p)$, and the measure of association is an *odds ratio* (OR). Actually, the estimation is performed on a log scale, using logit (i.e., log odds) as the quantity being modeled. Logistic regression is the regression model of choice for case–control studies, but it is often used with other designs when the outcome is binary. The `logit` command displays coefficients on a logit scale, whereas `logistic` displays odds-ratio estimates. I show only the use of `logistic`.

The `lbw1.dta` dataset is from a case–control study: a group of 59 newborns with low birthweights ($< 2{,}500$ g) was compared with a random sample of 130 normal-weight newborns. This design means that the way the dataset was used in section 13.1 was not quite right. It is unclear what the combined study population represents. Please forgive that abuse of the data. In the dataset, the variable `low` identifies cases and controls. The distribution and coding of `low` is shown by `tab1`:

```
. use lbw1.dta, clear
(Hosmer & Lemeshow data)

. tab1 low

-> tabulation of low

birthweight |
      <2500g |      Freq.      Percent        Cum.
-------------+-----------------------------------
      0. No  |        130        68.78        68.78
      1. Yes |         59        31.22       100.00
-------------+-----------------------------------
       Total |        189       100.00
```

With a dichotomous outcome (birthweight $< 2{,}500$ g versus $\geq 2{,}500$ g), the appropriate measure of association in a case–control study is the odds ratio. `cc` (see section 12.2) calculates the association between maternal smoking and low birthweight:

```
. cc low smoke
                                                      Proportion
                  |   Exposed   Unexposed  |    Total    Exposed
------------------+------------------------+-----------------------
            Cases |        30          29  |       59     0.5085
         Controls |        44          86  |      130     0.3385
------------------+------------------------+-----------------------
            Total |        74         115  |      189     0.3915

                  |  Point estimate  |   [95% Conf. Interval]
------------------+------------------+------------------------
       Odds ratio |     2.021944     |   1.029092   3.965864 (exact)
   Attr. frac. ex.|     .5054264     |    .0282695   .7478481 (exact)
   Attr. frac. pop|     .2569965     |
------------------+------------------+------------------------
                    chi2(1) =      4.92  Pr>chi2 = 0.0265
```

The main result is an odds ratio of 2.02 (95% CI: $1.03, 3.97$). A logistic regression gives the same result; however, now the confidence interval is calculated by an approximate method:

```
. logistic low smoke

Logistic regression                             Number of obs   =        189
                                                LR chi2(1)      =       4.87
                                                Prob > chi2     =     0.0274
Log likelihood =  -114.9023                     Pseudo R2       =     0.0207

-------------+----------------------------------------------------------------
         low | Odds Ratio   Std. Err.      z    P>|z|     [95% Conf. Interval]
-------------+----------------------------------------------------------------
       smoke |  2.021944    .6462912     2.20   0.028     1.080668    3.783083
-------------+----------------------------------------------------------------
```

In the output from logistic, the pseudo R^2 has no simple interpretation. Note that logistic's confidence intervals are constructed, not from the standard error displayed by logistic, but via a transformation of the model fit in the log scale. To see the "real" model fit, use the logit command:

```
. logit low smoke
```
(*output omitted*)

low	Coef.	Std. Err.	z	P>|z|	[95% Conf. Interval]	
smoke	.7040592	.3196386	2.20	0.028	.0775791	1.330539
_cons	-1.087051	.2147299	-5.06	0.000	-1.507914	-.6661886

As with linear regression, you can include continuous and categorical predictors and interactions:

```
. xi: logistic low i.smoke*i.race lwt
```

```
i.smoke            _Ismoke_0-1         (naturally coded; _Ismoke_0 omitted)
i.race             _Irace_1-3          (naturally coded; _Irace_1 omitted)
i.smoke*i.race     _IsmoXrac_#_#       (coded as above)
```

```
Logistic regression                            Number of obs    =        189
                                               LR chi2(6)       =      22.05
                                               Prob > chi2      =     0.0012
Log likelihood = -106.31314                    Pseudo R2        =     0.0939
```

low	Odds Ratio	Std. Err.	z	P>|z|	[95% Conf. Interval]	
_Ismoke_1	5.007368	3.030979	2.66	0.008	1.528882	16.40005
_Irace_2	5.100862	3.897479	2.13	0.033	1.140921	22.80508
_Irace_3	4.615637	2.790839	2.53	0.011	1.411087	15.09766
IsmoXrac~2	.6488813	.6833357	-0.41	0.681	.0823695	5.111684
IsmoXrac~3	.2572416	.2307854	-1.51	0.130	.0443284	1.492796
lwt	.9876706	.006333	-1.93	0.053	.9753359	1.000161

When controlling for prepregnancy weight (lwt), the association between smoking and low birthweight was OR = 5.007 for white women. For black women, it was 5.007 × 0.649 = 3.25, and for women of other race it was 5.007 × 0.257 = 1.29. For nonsmoking black women versus nonsmoking white women, the odds ratio was 5.10; for smoking women, the corresponding odds ratio was 5.101 × 0.649 = 3.31. You can estimate the odds ratio with the confidence interval for any combination of predictors by running the lincom command after logistic (see [R] **lincom**). The commands corresponding to the above calculations are

```
. lincom _Ismoke_1 + _IsmoXrac_1_2

 ( 1)  _Ismoke_1 + _IsmoXrac_1_2 = 0
```

low	Odds Ratio	Std. Err.	z	P>|z|	[95% Conf. Interval]	
(1)	3.249187	2.793182	1.37	0.170	.6026074	17.51923

```
. lincom _Ismoke_1 + _IsmoXrac_1_3

 ( 1)  _Ismoke_1 + _IsmoXrac_1_3 = 0
```

low	Odds Ratio	Std. Err.	z	P>|z|	[95% Conf. Interval]	
(1)	1.288103	.8533323	0.38	0.702	.3516037	4.718977

```
. lincom _Irace_2 + _IsmoXrac_1_2

 ( 1)  _Irace_2 + _IsmoXrac_1_2 = 0
```

low	Odds Ratio	Std. Err.	z	P>|z|	[95% Conf. Interval]	
(1)	3.309854	2.430699	1.63	0.103	.7846956	13.961

Concerning the continuous predictor `lwt` (mother's prepregnancy weight), the coefficient (0.9876706) is the odds ratio for low birthweight per pound of difference in maternal weight. If you want to express this per 50 lb. of difference in maternal weight, the corresponding odds ratio is $0.9876706^{50} = 0.54$. The confidence interval should be treated the same way. `lincom` gives the same result:

```
. lincom 50*lwt

 ( 1)  50 lwt = 0
```

low	Odds Ratio	Std. Err.	z	P>|z|	[95% Conf. Interval]	
(1)	.5377815	.1724135	-1.93	0.053	.286886	1.008097

You can use `predict` after `logistic` to obtain the predicted probability of the outcome for each observation; see [R] **predict**.

```
. xi: logistic low i.smoke i.race
i.smoke        _Ismoke_0-1      (naturally coded; _Ismoke_0 omitted)
i.race         _Irace_1-3       (naturally coded; _Irace_1 omitted)

Logistic regression                       Number of obs   =        189
                                          LR chi2(3)      =      14.70
                                          Prob > chi2     =     0.0021
Log likelihood = -109.98736               Pseudo R2       =     0.0626
```

low	Odds Ratio	Std. Err.	z	P>|z|	[95% Conf. Interval]	
_Ismoke_1	3.052631	1.12711	3.02	0.003	1.480433	6.294481
_Irace_2	2.956742	1.448758	2.21	0.027	1.131717	7.724832
_Irace_3	3.030001	1.212926	2.77	0.006	1.382618	6.640233

```
. predict plow if e(sample)
(option p assumed; Pr(low))
. table smoke, by(race) c(mean low mean plow) format(%8.4f) stubwidth(18)
```

race and smoked during pregnancy	mean(low)	mean(plow)
1. white		
0. No	0.0909	0.1370
1. Yes	0.3654	0.3264
2. black		
0. No	0.3125	0.3194
1. Yes	0.6000	0.5889
3. other		
0. No	0.3636	0.3248
1. Yes	0.4167	0.5948

low is the mean of the 0/1-coded variable, i.e., the observed proportion with low birth-weight, and plow is the probability predicted from the regression model for the combination of predictors in each observation. A different model would give different predicted probabilities. Although the observed and predicted probabilities from a case–control study give no meaning beyond the study population, we can compare them.

You could also let adjust (see section 13.1) produce the predicted probabilities; use the pr option:

```
. adjust, by(race smoke) pr
```

Dependent variable: low   Command: logistic
Variables left as is: _Ismoke_1, _Irace_2, _Irace_3

race	smoked during pregnancy	
	0. No	1. Yes
1. white	.136988	.326395
2. black	.319417	.588932
3. other	.324761	.594844

Key: Probability

For a goodness-of-fit test, we use estat gof after logistic (see [R] **logistic postestimation**). There are six different exposure combinations. The goodness-of-fit test leads us to accept the model:

```
. estat gof
```

Logistic model for low, goodness-of-fit test

```
        number of observations =       189
number of covariate patterns =         6
               Pearson chi2(2) =      3.12
                   Prob > chi2 =    0.2103
```

If there were many different exposure combinations, a better choice probably would be to use the Hosmer–Lemeshow goodness-of-fit test. We must choose the number of groups:

```
. estat gof, group(10)
```

Unlike regress and logit, logistic does not display a constant (intercept). This omission is sensible for case–control studies where the proportion of cases reflects the study design rather than any true prevalence. In other cases, you may want to see the constant (baseline odds; odds when all predictors are zero). To obtain that, use lincom immediately after logistic:

```
. lincom _cons

 ( 1)  _cons = 0
```

low	Odds Ratio	Std. Err.	z	P>|z|	[95% Conf. Interval]	
(1)	.1587319	.0560107	-5.22	0.000	.0794889	.3169727

Despite the header text, 0.159 is not an odds ratio but the baseline odds (the odds for the outcome when all predictors are zero)—in this example, the odds for low birthweight among white nonsmokers. The corresponding probability is $0.159/(1 + 0.159) = 13.7\%$. Remember, however, that this was a case–control study, so you cannot generalize absolute risks outside the study population.

For small sample sizes, logistic's maximum likelihood estimation can perform poorly; exlogistic is an exact alternative. For a description of the statistical principles, see Metha and Patel (1995). exlogistic is computationally intensive, and if you encounter problems, you need to study the help file or [R] **exlogistic**. In the following command, the condvars() option specifies variables whose parameter estimates are not of interest. This saves computer time and memory requirements. The nolog option prevents the display of the enumeration log, which can be quite extensive. The estimate is not very different from that found by the logistic analysis.

```
. exlogistic low smoke, condvars(race) nolog
```

Exact logistic regression

```
                                           Number of obs =       189
```

low	Odds Ratio	Suff.	2*Pr(Suff.)	[95% Conf. Interval]	
smoke	3.018679	30	0.0033	1.404664	6.745374

13.3   Other regression models

Variations and alternatives to logistic regression

The two commands `logistic` and `logit` (see [R] **logit**) do the same thing. The only difference is that `logit` displays the original coefficients, whereas `logistic` displays the exponentially transformed coefficients, or odds ratios. `exlogistic` performs an "exact" logistic regression. Do not use it with many observations as you will run out of memory and/or patience.

If the outcome of interest is not binary but may take several values, there are a few variations to logistic regression. If the outcome variable is ordinal, as in poor/average/good/excellent, see [R] **ologit** (ordered logit estimation). If the outcome variable is nominal with no natural rank order, as in Africa/Australia/Asia/Europe, etc., see [R] **mlogit** (multinomial or polytomous logistic regression). For matched case–control data, use `clogit` to perform a conditional logistic regression; see section 13.4.

Logistic regression corresponds directly to the case–control design, with odds ratios as the measure of association, but it is often used to analyze cohort data where relative risk is the "natural" measure of association. Binomial regression with the `binreg` command estimates relative risks; see [R] **binreg** and the short example in section 12.1.

Other models

Cox regression and Poisson regression are presented in chapter 14 on survival analysis.

There is a general engine behind most regression models in Stata: generalized linear models. The specific regression commands are modifications to these models. If you are curious, see [R] **glm**. To get an impression of the possibilities, you might take a look at the subject table in the *Quick Reference and Index*. In this chapter, I presented only the analyses most often used in health research.

13.4   Analyzing complex design data

For a nontechnical introduction to analyzing complex design data, I recommend reading chapter 5 in Campbell (2006) or chapters 21 and 30–31 in Kirkwood and Sterne (2003). I will mention two examples: matched case–control studies and repeated observations.

Matched case–control studies: Conditional logistic regression

In matched case–control data, we cannot ignore the matching criterion; it must be included in the analysis. In section 12.2, we used the `mcc` command to analyze 1:1 matched case–control data and saw that the principle is stratification by a variable identifying each matched set. Conditional logistic regression is the corresponding regression model and is performed with the `clogit` command; see [R] **clogit**. `clogit` is not restricted to 1:1 matched datasets. There can be any matching ratio, and the ratios may vary between the matched sets.

The `lowbirth.dta` dataset presented in section 12.2 consisted of 56 pairs of women, matched on age. In each pair, the case woman gave birth to a low-weight child, the control woman to a normal-weight child:

```
. webuse lowbirth.dta, clear
(Applied Logistic Regression, Hosmer & Lemeshow)

. codebook, compact

Variable   Obs Unique      Mean  Min  Max  Label

pairid     112     56      28.5    1   56  Case-control pair id
low        112      2        .5    0    1  Baby has low birthweight
age        112     20      22.5   14   34  Age of mother
lwt        112     57  127.1696   80  241  Mother's last menstrual weight
smoke      112      2  .4107143    0    1  Mother smoked during pregnancy
ptd        112      2  .2232143    0    1  Mother had previous preterm baby
ht         112      2  .0892857    0    1  Mother has hypertension
ui         112      2  .1785714    0    1  Uterine irritability
race1      112      2  .3928571    0    1  mother is white
race2      112      2    .1875     0    1  mother is black
race3      112      2  .4196429    0    1  mother is other
```

We want to estimate the effect of smoking, race, and age on the risk of low birthweight. Dummy variables for race are already included in the dataset. You must specify the matching-set identifier in the `group()` option. The `or` option displays odds ratios rather than the original coefficients:

```
. clogit low smoke race2 race3 age, group(pairid) or nolog
note: age omitted because of no within-group variance.
Conditional (fixed-effects) logistic regression   Number of obs   =       112
                                                  LR chi2(3)      =      8.44
                                                  Prob > chi2     =    0.0378
Log likelihood =  -34.59838                       Pseudo R2       =    0.1087
```

low	Odds Ratio	Std. Err.	z	P>|z|	[95% Conf. Interval]	
smoke	3.710822	1.849868	2.63	0.009	1.396822	9.858239
race2	1.380827	.8134253	0.55	0.584	.4352195	4.380966
race3	1.888002	.9757448	1.23	0.219	.6856305	5.19894

Interpreting the output is straightforward, just like with logistic regression. `clogit` dropped the matching criterion `age` from the analysis. When you match, you cannot possibly study the effect of the matching criteria.

`exlogistic` (see section 13.2) can be used for exact conditional logistic regression. The command corresponding to the above would be the following:

```
. exlogistic low smoke race2 race3, group(pairid) nolog
Exact logistic regression                        Number of obs       =         112
Group variable: pairid                           Number of groups    =          56

                                                 Obs per group: min  =           2
                                                                avg  =         2.0
                                                                max  =           2

                                                 Model score         =     7.91836
                                                 Pr >= score         =      0.0417
```

low	Odds Ratio	Suff.	2*Pr(Suff.)	[95% Conf. Interval]	
smoke	3.493165	30	0.0093	1.301029	11.07196
race2	1.348369	11	0.8139	.373617	5.048603
race3	1.859002	23	0.3170	.6426796	6.265291

Repeated and clustered observations

Hosmer and Lemeshow (2000) created a dataset consisting of 487 births among 188 women:

```
. use clslowbwt.dta

. codebook, compact
```

Variable	Obs	Unique	Mean	Min	Max	Label
id	487	188	93.44969	1	188	Mother id
birth	487	4	1.868583	1	4	Birth number
smoke	487	2	.4004107	0	1	Smoked during pregnancy
race	487	3	1.854209	1	3	Race
age	487	29	26.3963	14	43	Age of mother
lwt	487	131	142.6468	80	272	Prepregnancy weight
bwt	487	447	2840.115	798	5025	Birthweight, grams
low	487	2	.3100616	0	1	Birthweight < 2500g

A naïve analysis takes the 487 births as if they were just independent observations:

```
. logistic low age lwt smoke
Logistic regression                              Number of obs       =         487
                                                 LR chi2(3)          =       26.40
                                                 Prob > chi2         =      0.0000
Log likelihood = -288.32654                      Pseudo R2           =      0.0438
```

low	Odds Ratio	Std. Err.	z	P>|z|	[95% Conf. Interval]	
age	1.048515	.0196192	2.53	0.011	1.010759	1.087682
lwt	.9914686	.0034807	-2.44	0.015	.9846699	.9983143
smoke	2.235806	.4522966	3.98	0.000	1.503968	3.323759

But it is obvious that we do not have independent observations; the birthweights of siblings are correlated, and women have different tendencies to have children with a low birthweight. These different tendencies cannot be observed directly but are reflected in the data. Analyzing the data as if we had 487 independent observations leads to an exaggeration of the statistical precision, with standard errors that are too small and confidence intervals that are too narrow.

This is a common situation in health research: women may have more than one child, most people have two legs, and we have up to 32 teeth. The general principle for analyzing these data is to consider the woman, not the births, to be the primary sampling unit (PSU). You can do this by using the vce(cluster *clustvar*) option.

```
. logistic low age lwt smoke, vce(cluster id)

Logistic regression                             Number of obs   =        487
                                                Wald chi2(3)    =      12.26
                                                Prob > chi2     =     0.0065
Log pseudolikelihood = -288.32654               Pseudo R2       =     0.0438

                              (standard errors adjusted for clustering on id)

             |              Robust
         low | Odds Ratio  Std. Err.      z    P>|z|     [95% Conf. Interval]
-------------+----------------------------------------------------------------
         age |   1.048515   .0239779     2.07   0.038     1.002557    1.09658
         lwt |   .9914686   .0043187    -1.97   0.049     .9830403   .9999693
       smoke |   2.235806   .6386586     2.82   0.005     1.277286   3.913633
```

Comparing the two analyses, the point estimates are the same, but the standard errors increased and the confidence intervals became wider. For more information, see [U] **20.15 Obtaining robust variance estimates**.

Stata has a family of commands for analyzing survey data, which are described in the *Survey Data Reference Manual*. One common property of surveys is cluster sampling. Here it corresponds to the women being the PSU. Before analysis, you must organize the data by using the svyset command:

```
. svyset id
      pweight: <none>
          VCE: linearized
  Single unit: missing
    Strata 1: <one>
        SU 1: id
       FPC 1: <zero>

. svy: logistic low age lwt smoke
(running logistic on estimation sample)

Survey: Logistic regression

Number of strata   =          1             Number of obs     =        487
Number of PSUs     =        188             Population size   =        487
                                            Design df         =        187
                                            F(   3,    185)   =       4.04
                                            Prob > F          =     0.0082

             |            Linearized
         low | Odds Ratio  Std. Err.      t    P>|t|     [95% Conf. Interval]
-------------+----------------------------------------------------------------
         age |   1.048515   .0239779     2.07   0.040     1.002264     1.0969
         lwt |   .9914686   .0043187    -1.97   0.051     .9829856   1.000025
       smoke |   2.235806   .6386586     2.82   0.005     1.272636   3.927931
```

The result is close to what we found with `logistic` with the `vce(cluster` *clustvar*`)` option. The `svy:` prefix allows you to analyze complex sampling schemes, such as sampling of school classes, and then sampling of children within each class.

The `xt` family of commands is designed for panel data (repeated observations in a panel of study objects); see the *Longitudinal/Panel-Data Reference Manual*. Below I show a population-averaged model with options pa and `vce(robust)`. `xtlogit` gives the following result:

```
. xtset id
       panel variable:  id (unbalanced)

. xtlogit low age lwt smoke, or pa vce(robust) nolog

GEE population-averaged model              Number of obs      =        487
Group variable:                        id  Number of groups   =        188
Link:                               logit  Obs per group: min =          2
Family:                          binomial                 avg =        2.6
Correlation:                 exchangeable                 max =          4
                                           Wald chi2(3)       =      13.49
Scale parameter:                        1  Prob > chi2        =     0.0037

                              (Std. Err.  adjusted for clustering on id)
```

| | | Semi-robust | | | |
low	Odds Ratio	Std. Err.	z	P>|z|	[95% Conf. Interval]
age	1.061538	.0210929	3.01	0.003	1.020991	1.103695
lwt	.990815	.0040732	-2.24	0.025	.9828638	.9988305
smoke	2.014735	.5701286	2.48	0.013	1.157032	3.50825

The result differs a bit from what we saw before, but I cannot tell you which is the better choice. The `xt` commands also allow random-effects models, but they are beyond the scope of this book; see Campbell (2006), Dupont (2002), Kirkwood and Sterne (2003), and Hosmer and Lemeshow (2000) for discussions of the merits and weaknesses of different models. The examples in this section used logistic regression, but the principles apply in general: with complex data structures, such as those due to cluster sampling or repeated observations within individuals, the standard models are not valid. It might be a good idea to seek expert advice before you begin designing a study.

14 Incidence, mortality, and survival

14.1 Incidence and mortality

Incidence rates

An incidence rate is estimated by dividing the number of events by the corresponding time at risk. We use the compliance1.dta dataset, which has data on 555 men aged 64–73 years who were invited to a screening trial for abdominal aortic aneurysms and were monitored for up to 6 years after randomization; see Lindholt et al. 2005. These data concern a subset of the invited group only; data have been modified to conceal the identity of individuals. We have information on deaths, date of randomization (randate), and date of observation end (enddate). In codebook, the dates are not displayed with a date format but with their numeric value. For information about date variables, see section 5.5.

```
. cd C:\docs\ishr2
c:\docs\ishr2

. use compliance1.dta
(Compliance with invitation to a screening program)

. codebook, compact

Variable   Obs Unique      Mean    Min    Max  Label

id         555    555  6199.575     30  12630  Person number
particip   555      2   .7405405     0      1  Participated
birthdate  555    508  -12484.96 -14235  -9502  Date of birth
randate    555     12   12707.7   12512  14122  Date of randomization
enddate    555    101  14441.18   12597  14609  Date of last observation
died       555      2   .1855856     0      1  Died
```

From the dates, we want to calculate the time at risk in years (risktime), the age at randomization (ranage), this age in 2-year groups (ranagr), and the age at the end of observation (endage). These new variables are saved in compliance2.dta. The stset command will be explained in section 14.2.

```
                     ─────────── gen_compliance2.do ───────────
* gen_compliance2.do

cd C:\docs\ishr2
use compliance1.dta

generate risktime=(enddate-randate)/365.25
generate ranage=(randate-birthdate)/365.25
generate endage=(enddate-birthdate)/365.25
generate ranagr=2*int(ranage/2)

label variable risktime "Time at risk"
label variable ranage "Age at randomization"
label variable endage "Age at observation end"
label variable ranagr "Age group at randomization"
label define ranagr 64 "64-65" 66 "66-67" 68 "68-69" 70 "70-71" 72 "72-73"
label values ranagr ranagr

stset risktime, failure(died==1) id(id)

label data "Compliance data -stset- from randomization"
save compliance2.dta
```

We can obtain the number of deaths and the time at risk by typing

```
. use compliance2.dta
(Compliance data -stset- from randomization)

. tabstat died risktime, stat(sum)

    stats │      died  risktime
──────────┼────────────────────
      sum │       103  2634.032
```

From the 103 deaths and the time at risk of 2,634 years, we can estimate the mortality rate by calculating $103/2634$ years $= 0.039$ deaths per year, or 39 deaths per 1,000 years. ci estimates the rate and calculates the exact Poisson confidence interval; it is 32 to 47 deaths per 1,000 years:

```
. ci died, exposure(risktime) poisson

                                               ── Poisson Exact ──
    Variable │  Exposure      Mean    Std. Err.    [95% Conf. Interval]
─────────────┼──────────────────────────────────────────────────────────
        died │  2634.032   .0391036    .003853     .0319176    .0474244
```

If we know the number of deaths and time at risk, we can also use the immediate command cii; see section 10.5.

If we have stset the data (see section 14.2), we can obtain an overview of events, time at risk, and incidence rates by stptime. The dd() option lets us decide the number of decimals to display.

```
. stptime, by(particip) per(1000) dd(4)

         failure _d:  died == 1
   analysis time _t:  risktime
                 id:  id
```

particip	person-time	failures	rate	[95% Conf. Interval]	
0. No	622.1164	42	67.5115	49.8924	91.3526
1. Yes	2011.9151	61	30.3194	23.5904	38.9678
total	2634.0315	103	39.1036	32.2363	47.4338

We can also display the information for selected time intervals. The argument for the at() option is a numeric list; see section 4.3.

```
. stptime, by(particip) per(1000) dd(4) at(0(1)5)

         failure _d:  died == 1
   analysis time _t:  risktime
                 id:  id
```

particip	person-time	failures	rate	[95% Conf. Interval]	
0. No					
(0 - 1]	137.8782	12	87.0334	49.4271	153.2521
(1 - 2]	124.0424	8	64.4941	32.2533	128.9629
(2 - 3]	116.6441	5	42.8654	17.8418	102.9855
(3 - 4]	109.4901	6	54.7995	24.6193	121.9770
(4 - 5]	97.4237	9	92.3800	48.0667	177.5464
> 5	36.6379	2	54.5882	13.6524	218.2677
1. Yes					
(0 - 1]	408.8255	5	12.2302	5.0905	29.3833
(1 - 2]	390.9090	13	33.2558	19.3102	57.2728
(2 - 3]	374.6003	7	18.6866	8.9085	39.1971
(3 - 4]	356.4196	15	42.0852	25.3717	69.8086
(4 - 5]	331.5715	15	45.2391	27.2731	75.0401
> 5	149.5893	6	40.1098	18.0198	89.2796
total	2634.0315	103	39.1036	32.2363	47.4338

Comparing rates: Stratified analysis

We want to compare the overall mortality rates for those who accepted the screening offer with those who did not. The question is not whether screening for aneurysms affects overall mortality (aneurysms constitute only a small fraction of all deaths) but whether the general health of the participants differs from that of the nonparticipants.

However, mortality depends on age, and the tendency to accept a screening offer probably varies with age, too. To explore the association of participation and mortality with age, we can use tabstat:

```
. tabstat particip died, by(ranagr) format(%6.2f)
```

Summary statistics: mean
   by categories of: ranagr (Age group at randomization)

ranagr	particip	died
64-65	0.80	0.08
66-67	0.83	0.13
68-69	0.70	0.26
70-71	0.67	0.17
72-73	0.69	0.29
Total	0.74	0.19

particip and died are coded 0/1, so the mean (tabstat's default) displays the proportion of subjects who participated and died within the observation period. Participation clearly declines with age. We could test whether the decline is significant, but that is not the point: significantly or not, participation declines with age in our data, and that may confound the comparison of mortality between participants and nonparticipants. To study the participation–mortality association (incidence-rate ratio [IRR]), we use ir (see [ST] **epitab**). To adjust for age at randomization by stratification, we use ir with the by() option:

```
. ir died particip risktime, by(ranagr)
```

Age group at ran	IRR	[95% Conf. Interval]		M-H Weight	
64-65	.3140617	.0744762	1.513131	3.307495	(exact)
66-67	.4926495	.1420931	2.151985	3.341521	(exact)
68-69	.5236575	.228229	1.24793	8.088149	(exact)
70-71	.7504398	.2471127	2.512317	4.137178	(exact)
72-73	.4302365	.2117449	.8811187	12.27482	(exact)
Crude	.4490994	.2982485	.6820111		(exact)
M-H combined	.4913825	.3313807	.7286386		

Test of homogeneity (M-H)   chi2(4) =   1.34 Pr>chi2 = 0.8549

We can now see the crude mortality-rate ratio estimate (IRR = 0.45), as well as an age-adjusted estimate (IRR = 0.49; 95% CI: 0.33, 0.73). Adjusting for age thus somewhat reduced the contrast between participants and nonparticipants. The test of homogeneity (Pr = 0.85) tells us that there is no evidence of a different association by age (effect modification, interaction).

If we have stset our data (see section 14.2), we can obtain the same analysis by typing

```
. stir particip, by(ranagr)
```

The regression model corresponding to ir is poisson; here we adjust for age at randomization. No wonder that mortality increases with age; the association between participation and mortality is similar to what we found in the age-stratified analysis. Poisson regression is described in more detail in section 14.5.

```
. xi: poisson died particip i.ranagr, exposure(risktime) irr nolog
i.ranagr          _Iranagr_64-72      (naturally coded; _Iranagr_64 omitted)

Poisson regression                          Number of obs   =        555
                                            LR chi2(5)      =      32.23
                                            Prob > chi2     =     0.0000
Log likelihood = -338.40635                 Pseudo R2       =     0.0454
```

died	IRR	Std. Err.	z	P>|z|	[95% Conf. Interval]	
particip	.4889067	.0989234	-3.54	0.000	.3288496	.7268666
_Iranagr_66	1.447485	.599327	0.89	0.372	.6429489	3.258754
_Iranagr_68	2.679351	.9941403	2.66	0.008	1.294797	5.544437
_Iranagr_70	1.663297	.6732149	1.26	0.209	.7523992	3.67698
_Iranagr_72	3.238091	1.161152	3.28	0.001	1.60345	6.539172
risktime	(exposure)					

Here we stratified by age at the start of the observation period, but we can get more consistent results; see sections 14.3 and 14.5.

14.2   Survival analysis

In survival analysis, the key variable is the time until an event, such as death, recovery from a fracture, or the duration of the effect of a painkiller. Even if we lose sight of some persons during follow-up (censorings), we can still estimate the proportion of survivors until the end of follow-up, assuming that the risk of those censored does not differ from that of those still under observation. See any good biostatistical or epidemiological textbook, such as Kirkwood and Sterne (2003), for general principles. A more advanced book is Hosmer, Lemeshow, and May (2008). Stata-specific texts are the *Survival Analysis and Epidemiological Tables Reference Manual* and Cleves et al. (2008).

Life table method

The classical method of survival analysis is the life table or actuarial method. ltable (see [ST] **ltable**) evaluates the survivor function at selected points in time; it also displays the number of persons at risk and the number of events (deaths) and censorings (lost). Although theoretically inferior to the Kaplan–Meier survival estimate (see later in this section), the result comes close if the time intervals are reasonably short. If you can only locate events within prespecified time intervals, you may prefer this method. An example might be persons examined for a disease with annual intervals; you know in which interval the disease occurred but not when.

(Continued on next page)

```
. use compliance2.dta
(Compliance data -stset- from randomization)

. ltable risktime died, intervals(0(1)5) by(particip)
```

	Interval	Beg. Total	Deaths	Lost	Survival	Std. Error	[95% Conf. Int.]	
0. No								
0	1	144	12	0	0.9167	0.0230	0.8579	0.9518
1	2	132	8	5	0.8600	0.0290	0.7915	0.9074
2	3	119	5	1	0.8238	0.0320	0.7503	0.8773
3	4	113	6	3	0.7794	0.0350	0.7012	0.8395
4	5	104	9	3	0.7110	0.0387	0.6273	0.7792
5	.	92	2	90	0.6807	0.0425	0.5893	0.7560
1. Yes								
0	1	411	5	0	0.9878	0.0054	0.9710	0.9949
1	2	406	13	13	0.9557	0.0102	0.9306	0.9719
2	3	380	7	4	0.9380	0.0120	0.9096	0.9577
3	4	369	15	9	0.8994	0.0151	0.8654	0.9252
4	5	345	15	8	0.8598	0.0176	0.8213	0.8906
5	.	322	6	316	0.8284	0.0211	0.7824	0.8655

After 5 years (at the end of interval 4–5), the proportion surviving was 71% among nonparticipants and 86% among participants.

Preparations for survival analysis: The stset command

To prepare for survival analysis (other than with ltable), we use the stset command; see [ST] **stset**. The stset command was included in gen_compliance2.do, section 14.1, and resulted in this output:

```
. stset risktime, failure(died==1) id(id)

               id:  id
    failure event:  died == 1
obs. time interval:  (risktime[_n-1], risktime]
 exit on or before:  failure

         555  total obs.
           0  exclusions

         555  obs. remaining, representing
         555  subjects
         103  failures in single failure-per-subject data
    2634.032  total analysis time at risk, at risk from t =        0
                          earliest observed entry t =        0
                           last observed exit t =  5.741273
```

In the stset command, we defined risktime (time from randomization to end of observation) as the time variable and the code 1 for died (failure, in this case death, as opposed to censored at the end of observation). We do not really need the id() option now, but we will need it later (see stsplit, section 14.4). The stset output tells us, as we have already seen, that we have 555 observations with 103 failures and a total time at risk of 2,634 years. After we run stset, the dataset includes the following variables:

```
. codebook, compact

Variable    Obs Unique      Mean      Min      Max  Label

id          555    555   6199.575       30    12630  Person number
particip    555      2   .7405405        0        1  Participated
birthdate   555    508  -12484.96   -14235    -9502  Date of birth
randate     555     12    12707.7    12512    14122  Date of randomization
enddate     555    101   14441.18    12597    14609  Date of last observation
died        555      2   .1855856        0        1  Died
risktime    555    112   4.746003  .1670089  5.741273  Time at risk
ranage      555    494   68.97373  64.27105  73.79877  Age at randomization
endage      555    508   73.71974  65.51403  78.97057  Age at observation end
ranagr      555      5   67.94595       64       72  Age group at randomization
_st         555      1          1        1        1
_d          555      2   .1855856        0        1
_t          555    112   4.746003  .1670089  5.741273
_t0         555      1          0        0        0
```

stset created four new variables, which are used for a number of analyses:

_st   The code 1 means that the observation has valid survival information, such as positive time at risk and a defined status (_d) at observation end.

_d   The code 0 means censoring, and 1 means failure; here it is identical with died.

_t   The time at observation end; here it is identical with risktime.

_t0   The time at observation start; here it is 0 for everyone.

Once the data are stset, you can easily perform several survival analyses.

The Kaplan–Meier survivor function

sts list lets us tabulate the Kaplan–Meier survivor function; see [ST] **sts list**. Without the at() option, we would get a line for each event. The failure option would tabulate 1 − survival instead of survival.

(Continued on next page)

```
. sts list, by(particip) at(0(1)5)

        failure _d:  died == 1
   analysis time _t:  risktime
                id:  id

                Beg.                    Survivor      Std.
     Time       Total      Fail        Function      Error      [95% Conf. Int.]
```

	Time	Beg. Total	Fail	Survivor Function	Std. Error	[95% Conf. Int.]	
0. No							
	0	0	0	1.0000	.	.	.
	1	133	12	0.9167	0.0230	0.8579	0.9518
	2	120	8	0.8597	0.0291	0.7910	0.9071
	3	114	5	0.8233	0.0321	0.7497	0.8770
	4	105	6	0.7784	0.0352	0.6998	0.8387
	5	93	9	0.7096	0.0388	0.6256	0.7781
1. Yes							
	0	0	0	1.0000	.	.	.
	1	407	5	0.9878	0.0054	0.9710	0.9949
	2	381	13	0.9556	0.0102	0.9304	0.9718
	3	370	7	0.9378	0.0120	0.9093	0.9576
	4	346	15	0.8990	0.0152	0.8648	0.9249
	5	323	15	0.8593	0.0176	0.8207	0.8902

```
Note:  survivor function is calculated over full data and evaluated at
       indicated times; it is not calculated from aggregates shown at left.
```

To see the actual number at risk, e.g., after 1 year, use ltable. The numbers displayed by sts list under the heading Beg. Total are slightly different (they are the number at risk at the time of the preceding failure event).

To create a graph with a Kaplan–Meier plot for participants and nonparticipants, the basic command is this simple (the full do-file to create figure 14.1 is available at this book's web site):

```
. sts graph, by(particip)
```

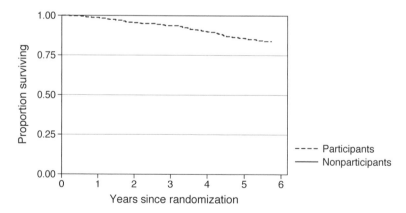

Figure 14.1. Kaplan–Meier plots for two groups

With most subjects surviving, most of the plot area in figure 14.1 is empty. Pocock, Clayton, and Altman (2002) recommend plotting the cumulative incidence proportion (1 − survival) instead. The `failure` option allows that, as shown in the following command and figure 14.2. They also recommend stating the number still at risk at selected points in time. These numbers are generated by the `risktable` option. The `ylabel()` option defines the labels at the y axis. Without it, the y axis would still span from 0 to 1. Here I show the basic command; the full do-file to create figure 14.2 is available at this book's web site:

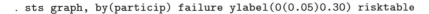

. sts graph, by(particip) failure ylabel(0(0.05)0.30) risktable

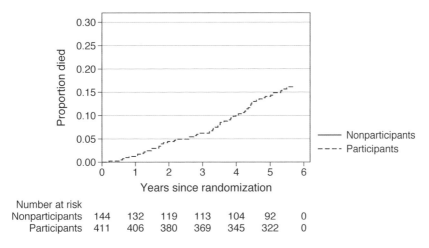

Figure 14.2. Kaplan–Meier plots of cumulative incidence proportion (1 – survival)

Log-rank test

The log-rank test compares the observed and expected distribution of events between two or more groups; see [ST] **sts test**.

```
. sts test particip

        failure _d:  died == 1
   analysis time _t:  risktime
                id:  id

Log-rank test for equality of survivor functions
```

particip	Events observed	Events expected
0. No	42	24.23
1. Yes	61	78.77
Total	103	103.00

```
                chi2(1) =      17.06
                Pr>chi2 =     0.0000
```

The test can be stratified. Here it is stratified by age at randomization:

```
. sts test particip, strata(ranagr)

        failure _d:  died == 1
   analysis time _t:  risktime
                id:  id

Stratified log-rank test for equality of survivor functions

              |      Events         Events
   particip   |    observed     expected(*)
--------------+--------------------------------
   0. No      |          42           26.14
   1. Yes     |          61           76.86
--------------+--------------------------------
   Total      |         103          103.00

(*) sum over calculations within ranagr

              chi2(1) =        13.09
              Pr>chi2 =       0.0003
```

Several alternative tests are available; see [ST] **sts test**.

14.3 Cox regression

Proportional hazards model

Cox proportional hazards regression estimates hazard ratios. For all practical purposes, they can be interpreted as incidence-rate ratios. Once the data are stset, we can just call stcox with the predictors; see [ST] **stcox**. Here we want to see the association with participation while controlling for age at randomization. The schoenfeld() and basesurv() options are necessary for some of the following analyses (estat phtest and stcurve).

```
. use compliance2.dta
(Compliance data -stset- from randomization)

. xi: stcox particip i.ranagr, schoenfeld(sch*) basesurv(s) nolog
i.ranagr            _Iranagr_64-72      (naturally coded; _Iranagr_64 omitted)

        failure _d:  died == 1
  analysis time _t:  risktime
               id:  id

Cox regression -- Breslow method for ties

No. of subjects =         555              Number of obs    =         555
No. of failures =         103
Time at risk    =  2634.031508
                                           LR chi2(5)       =       31.68
Log likelihood  =   -617.90439             Prob > chi2      =      0.0000
```

_t	Haz. Ratio	Std. Err.	z	P>|z|	[95% Conf.	Interval]
particip	.4844013	.0981015	-3.58	0.000	.325701	.7204295
_Iranagr_66	1.389571	.5758334	0.79	0.427	.6168016	3.130514
_Iranagr_68	2.576273	.9569668	2.55	0.011	1.243969	5.335487
_Iranagr_70	1.58765	.6435182	1.14	0.254	.7173637	3.513744
_Iranagr_72	3.116361	1.120295	3.16	0.002	1.540461	6.304414

The result is similar to that from the corresponding Poisson regression (section 14.1), and the overall interpretation is the same.

The proportional-hazards requirement means that the hazard ratio or incidence-rate ratio is constant over the time of follow-up. Looking at figure 14.2, we get the impression that during the first year after randomization, the mortality among nonparticipants is much higher than that among participants, while the difference is less marked later (this outcome was actually expected: current ill health may reduce a subject's ability and motivation to participate in a preventive examination). For a graphical assessment of the requirement, we use stphplot (see [ST] **stcox diagnostics**) as shown in figure 14.3:

(Continued on next page)

```
. stphplot, by(particip)
```

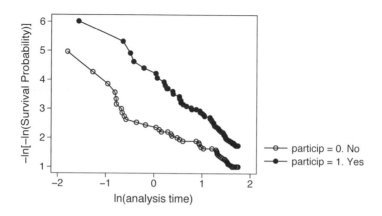

Figure 14.3. Assessment of the proportional-hazards requirement with stphplot

When the proportional-hazards requirement is fulfilled, the lines are roughly parallel; here we may be in doubt as to whether the departure is important. We can test this question formally by running estat phtest (see [ST] **stcox postestimation**) after stcox with the schoenfeld() option. Here we found it was far from significant, so we can accept the proportional-hazards assumption:

```
. estat phtest
    Test of proportional hazards assumption

    Time:   Time
```

	chi2	df	Prob>chi2
global test	3.88	5	0.5667

If we accept the proportional-hazards assumption, we can make a graph that corresponds to the assumption, using stcurve after stcox with the basesurv() option (figure 14.4):

```
. stcurve, survival at1(particip=0) at2(particip=1)
> ylabel(.7(.05)1, grid)
```

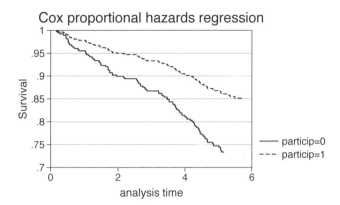

Figure 14.4. Estimated survival curves, based on the proportional-hazards assumption

The graph depends on the proportional-hazards assumption, but it does not tell us whether the assumption is true.

Using age as the time axis (delayed entry)

Until now, we have analyzed data along a time axis, starting when the subject entered the study (the date of randomization). But the subjects entered the study at different ages, and because age is a strong predictor of mortality, it should be taken into account. We have done that by stratifying or adjusting by the age at randomization, but we can make a more consistent adjustment by using age as the time axis. To do that, we must stset the data again, using the age at observation start (ranage) and end (endage):

```
────────────── gen_compliance3.do ──────────────
* gen_compliance3.do

cd C:\docs\ishr2
use compliance2.dta

stset endage, enter(time ranage) failure(died==1) id(id)

label data "Compliance data stset with age as time axis"
save compliance3.dta, replace
```

The output from `stset` follows:

```
. stset endage, enter(time ranage) failure(died==1) id(id)

              id:  id
   failure event:  died == 1
obs. time interval:  (endage[_n-1], endage]
 enter on or after:  time ranage
 exit on or before:  failure
─────────────────────────────────────────────────────────────────────────
        555  total obs.
          0  exclusions
─────────────────────────────────────────────────────────────────────────
        555  obs. remaining, representing
        555  subjects
        103  failures in single failure-per-subject data
   2634.031  total analysis time at risk, at risk from t =          0
                              earliest observed entry t =   64.27105
                                 last observed exit t =   78.97057
```

We defined `ranage` as the entry time (`_t0`) and `endage` as the end of the observation time (`_t`). The number of events and the time at risk remain unchanged, but the key variables now are as follows:

```
. use compliance3.dta, clear
(Compliance data stset with age as time axis)

. codebook ranage endage _*, compact

Variable    Obs Unique     Mean      Min      Max  Label
─────────────────────────────────────────────────────────────────────────
ranage      555    494  68.97373  64.27105  73.79877  Age at randomization
endage      555    508  73.71974  65.51403  78.97057  Age at observation end
_st         555      1         1         1         1
_d          555      2  .1855856         0         1
_t          555    508  73.71974  65.51403  78.97057
_t0         555    494  68.97373  64.27105  73.79877
─────────────────────────────────────────────────────────────────────────
```

To tabulate the survivor function with age as the time axis, we use `sts list` with the `at()` option; I use 2-year age groups:

```
. sts list, by(particip) at(64(2)80)

            failure _d:  died == 1
      analysis time _t:  endage
   enter on or after:    time ranage
                   id:   id
```

	Time	Beg. Total	Fail	Survivor Function	Std. Error	[95% Conf. Int.]	
0. No							
	64	0	0	1.0000	.	.	.
	66	23	1	0.9444	0.0540	0.6664	0.9920
	68	35	0	0.9444	0.0540	0.6664	0.9920
	70	52	8	0.7861	0.0682	0.6141	0.8880
	72	64	8	0.6856	0.0681	0.5314	0.7982
	74	82	8	0.6120	0.0656	0.4709	0.7260
	76	45	8	0.5441	0.0626	0.4142	0.6569
	78	18	9	0.3985	0.0625	0.2765	0.5175
	80	1	0	.	.	.	.
1. Yes							
	64	0	0	1.0000	.	.	.
	66	99	2	0.9779	0.0155	0.9143	0.9944
	68	165	3	0.9560	0.0197	0.8953	0.9819
	70	216	7	0.9208	0.0231	0.8610	0.9555
	72	194	7	0.8881	0.0254	0.8268	0.9286
	74	190	17	0.8129	0.0290	0.7480	0.8627
	76	119	13	0.7476	0.0320	0.6785	0.8041
	78	46	11	0.6433	0.0414	0.5558	0.7179
	80	1	1	.	.	.	.

```
Note:  survivor function is calculated over full data and evaluated at
       indicated times; it is not calculated from aggregates shown at left.
```

Now events are put in the age interval when they happened, and each individual's time at risk is distributed to several age intervals. With age as the time axis, the log-rank test is age adjusted:

```
. sts test particip

            failure _d:  died == 1
      analysis time _t:  endage
   enter on or after:    time ranage
                   id:   id
```

Log-rank test for equality of survivor functions

particip	Events observed	Events expected
0. No	42	26.01
1. Yes	61	76.99
Total	103	103.00

$$\text{chi2(1)} = 13.25$$
$$\text{Pr>chi2} = 0.0003$$

We can now make an age-adjusted Cox regression. With age as the time axis, we cannot study the effect of age itself, just as a stratified analysis does not let us see the effect of the stratification criterion:

```
. stcox particip, nolog

          failure _d:  died == 1
    analysis time _t:  endage
   enter on or after:  time ranage
                  id:  id

Cox regression -- Breslow method for ties

No. of subjects =            555          Number of obs   =         555
No. of failures =            103
Time at risk    =    2634.031448
                                          LR chi2(1)      =       11.95
Log likelihood  =    -539.34834           Prob > chi2     =      0.0005
```

_t	Haz. Ratio	Std. Err.	z	P>|z|	[95% Conf. Interval]
particip	.4875633	.0982525	-3.56	0.000	.3284725 .7237073

Compared with our previous attempts to adjust for age, the results are similar. Letting age be the time axis corresponds to a very fine stratification by age.

14.4 Reorganizing st data

stsplit

We can split an observation into several observations, each describing the experience within a shorter segment of time; see [ST] **stsplit**. We start with the compliance3.dta dataset created in section 14.3; it was stset with age as the time axis:

```
. use compliance3.dta
(Compliance data stset with age as time axis)

. codebook id _t0 _t risktime _d died, compact

Variable  Obs Unique      Mean        Min       Max  Label

id        555    555   6199.575         30     12630  Person number
_t0       555    494   68.97373   64.27105  73.79877
_t        555    508   73.71974   65.51403  78.97057
risktime  555    112   4.746003   .1670089  5.741273  Time at risk
_d        555      2   .1855856          0         1
died      555      2   .1855856          0         1  Died
```

For illustration, we can list two selected observations, one that was censored and one that ended in death:

```
. list id _t0 _t risktime _d died if id==249 | id==251
```

	id	_t0	_t	risktime	_d	died
8.	249	73.171799	78.40657	5.234771	0	0. No
9.	251	72.240929	76.035591	3.794661	1	1. Yes

The first person (id 249) had 5.23 years at risk, from age 73.17 until he was censored at age 78.41. The second person (id 251) had 3.79 years at risk, from age 72.24 until he died at age 76.04. With `stsplit`, we now split each observation in 2-year age groups:

```
_____ gen_compliance4.do _____
* gen_compliance4.do

cd C:\docs\ishr2
use compliance3.dta
stsplit age, at(64(2)80)

* risktime must be recalculated after splitting.
replace risktime = _t - _t0

label data "Compliance data stsplit 2-year age groups"
save compliance4.dta, replace
```

Now the dataset has been expanded to 1,901 observations, with deaths and time at risk allocated to the proper age intervals:

```
. codebook id _t0 _t risktime _d died age, compact

Variable     Obs Unique     Mean       Min        Max  Label

id          1901   555  6215.619        30       12630  Person number
_t0         1901   501  70.83873  64.27105          78
_t          1901   515  72.22433  65.51403    78.97057
risktime    1901   760  1.385603  .0013657           2  Time at risk
_d          1901     2   .054182         0           1
died         555     2  .1855856         0           1  Died
age         1901     8  70.53866        64          78
```

```
. sort id _t0
. list id _t0 _t risktime _d died if id==249 | id==251, sepby(id)
```

	id	_t0	_t	risktime	_d	died
27.	249	73.171799	74	.8282013	0	.
28.	249	74	76	2	0	.
29.	249	76	78	2	0	.
30.	249	78	78.40657	.4065704	0	0. No
31.	251	72.240929	74	1.759071	0	.
32.	251	74	76	2	0	.
33.	251	76	76.035591	.0355911	1	1. Yes

We can display the number of events and the time at risk for each age interval with `stptime`:

```
. stptime, by(age) per(1000) dd(4)

          failure _d:  died == 1
    analysis time _t:  endage
   enter on or after:  time ranage
                  id:  id
```

age	person-time	failures	rate	[95% Conf. Interval]	
64	129.6399	3	23.1410	7.4635	71.7503
66	307.9316	3	9.7424	3.1421	30.2071
68	465.4429	15	32.2274	19.4288	53.4569
70	507.2169	15	29.5731	17.8286	49.0543
72	529.0705	25	47.2527	31.9291	69.9305
74	437.0404	21	48.0505	31.3293	73.6962
76	220.8980	20	90.5395	58.4122	140.3371
78	36.7912	1	27.1804	3.8287	192.9555
total	2634.0314	103	39.1036	32.2363	47.4338

14.5 Poisson regression

As shown in section 14.1, Poisson is the regression model corresponding to a stratified analysis by `ir`. Think of the dataset as stratified by one or more criteria, each stratum including information on the number of events and the corresponding time at risk.

The `stsplit` dataset compliance4.dta, generated in section 14.4, is stratified by the variables `particip` (two categories) and `age` (eight categories). We can now perform a Poisson regression adjusted for age. The result is similar to that from the Cox regression in section 14.3: IRR $= 0.48$ (95% CI: $0.33, 0.72$).

```
. use compliance4.dta, clear
(Compliance data stsplit 2-year age groups)
. xi: poisson _d particip i.age, exposure(risktime) irr nolog
i.age            _Iage_64-78      (naturally coded; _Iage_64 omitted)

Poisson regression                        Number of obs   =       1901
                                          LR chi2(8)      =      37.53
                                          Prob > chi2     =     0.0000
Log likelihood = -464.45208               Pseudo R2       =     0.0388
```

_d	IRR	Std. Err.	z	P>|z|	[95% Conf. Interval]	
particip	.4834584	.0974273	-3.61	0.000	.3257044	.7176203
_Iage_66	.4220758	.3446237	-1.06	0.291	.0851897	2.091192
_Iage_68	1.376857	.8708156	0.51	0.613	.3985954	4.756036
_Iage_70	1.213949	.7680285	0.31	0.759	.3512947	4.194978
_Iage_72	1.883083	1.151588	1.03	0.301	.5679662	6.243332
_Iage_74	1.885421	1.165099	1.03	0.305	.5615737	6.330088
_Iage_76	3.619279	2.242606	2.08	0.038	1.074469	12.19131
_Iage_78	1.064129	1.22919	0.05	0.957	.1106014	10.23831
risktime	(exposure)					

The first variable in the command (`_d`) is the event variable; next follow the covariates, while the time at risk is specified in the `exposure()` option.

The same Poisson regression (but not a Cox regression) could also be performed on a collapsed dataset (on collapse, see section 9.6). The result is the same; below we list the collapsed dataset with 16 observations after having calculated the mortality rate.

```
. collapse (sum) risktime _d, by(particip age)
. generate mrate = _d/risktime
. list, sepby(particip)
```

	particip	age	risktime	_d	mrate
1.	0. No	64	22.85012	1	.0437634
2.	0. No	66	53.40452	0	0
3.	0. No	68	87.97673	8	.0909331
4.	0. No	70	119.1444	8	.0671454
5.	0. No	72	142.8953	8	.055985
6.	0. No	74	126.2738	8	.0633544
7.	0. No	76	58.84052	9	.1529558
8.	0. No	78	10.73101	0	0
9.	1. Yes	64	106.7898	2	.0187284
	(output omitted)				
16.	1. Yes	78	26.06023	1	.0383727

With few events, poisson's maximum likelihood estimation can perform poorly. An exact alternative is expoisson. It is computationally intensive, and if you encounter problems, you need to study the help file or [R] **expoisson**. The condvars() option specifies variables whose parameter estimates are not of interest; this saves computer time and memory requirements, but here we still needed to use the memory() option to request extra memory for the calculations. The estimate is not very different from that of the poisson analysis. Actually, the use of expoisson was hardly justified in this case. With many events, the estimates from poisson are valid.

```
. xi: expoisson _d particip, exposure(risktime) condvars(i.age) irr
> nolog memory(100m)
i.age            _Iage_64-78        (naturally coded; _Iage_64 omitted)

Exact Poisson regression
                                          Number of obs =        16
```

_d	IRR	Suff.	2*Pr(Suff.)	[95% Conf. Interval]	
particip	.4834584	61	0.0007	.3203509	.7357395
risktime	(exposure)				

14.6 Standardization

Standardization methods are examples of stratified analysis, but with weighting methods different from those of Mantel–Haenszel (see chapter 12). In *indirect standardization*, the incidence in the study population is compared with the incidence in a chosen reference population. Stratum weights are defined by the distribution of time at risk in the study population, and the result is expressed as standardized mortality ratio (SMR) or standardized incidence ratio (SIR). In *direct standardization*, the reference population is real or hypothetical; it is characterized by its relative age distribution, and standardized rates are calculated using the weights from the reference population.

Indirect standardization

A total of 192 Danish people had a certain operation between 1985 and 1996. They were monitored until they died or until 31 December 2004, whichever came first. The main information is recorded in oppatients1.dta:

```
. use oppatients1.dta
(Long term mortality after operation)

. codebook, compact

Variable   Obs Unique      Mean       Min       Max  Label

patid      192    192      96.5         1       192  Patient ID
sex        192      2  1.395833         1         2  Sex
bdate      192    192  -8319.198    -19533      4469  Date of birth
begdate    192    190  11561.14      9133     13514  Date of observation start
died       192      2  .2760417         0         1  Died
ddate       53     53   13169.7      9595     16426  Date of death
enddate    192     54  15534.36      9595     16436  Date of death/censoring
begage     192    192  54.42939   16.3258  83.35934  Age at observation start
endage     192    192  65.30749   32.76386  92.18069  Age at death/censoring
```

We want to express the prognosis after operation by comparing the patients' mortality with that of the general Danish population. The dk1991-95.dta dataset holds the age- and sex-specific mortality for Danes during 1991–95, and we use that as the reference:

```
. use dk1991-95.dta
(Data file created by EpiData based on dkk1991-95.rec)

. list, sepby(sex)
```

	sex	agegr	mrate
1.	1. male	0	.00666
2.	1. male	1	.00037
3.	1. male	5	.00021
4.	1. male	10	.00021
5.	1. male	15	.00063
	(output omitted)		
21.	1. male	95	.42985
22.	2. female	0	.0052
	(output omitted)		
38.	2. female	75	.04496
39.	2. female	80	.07604
40.	2. female	85	.1317
41.	2. female	90	.22301
42.	2. female	95	.3662

To proceed, we must `stset` the data, using age as the time axis (see section 14.2) and then `stsplit` the observations in age bands corresponding to the file containing the reference rates (see section 14.4). Finally, `merge` the reference mortality rates to the expanded dataset:

```
                        ─────────── gen_oppatients2.do ───────────
* gen_oppatients2.do

clear
cd C:\docs\ishr2
use oppatients1.dta

* -stset- data; age is time axis
stset endage, enter(time begage) failure(died==1) id(patid)

* split information in age bands (agegr)
  stsplit agegr, at(0 1 5(5)100)
  label variable agegr "Age band"

* Merge age- and sex-specific reference mortality rates to data
  sort sex agegr
  merge sex agegr using dk1991-95.dta
  drop if _merge<3       // Some age bands in the reference mortality rate file
  drop _merge            // had no match in the actual dataset; they are dropped

label data "Patient data, stsplit and merged with population rates"
save oppatients2.dta, replace
```

The merged dataset, `oppatients2.dta`, now includes 606 valid observations:

```
. use oppatients2.dta
(Patient data, stsplit and merged with population rates)

. codebook, compact

Variable   Obs Unique      Mean       Min       Max  Label

patid      606    192   89.02805        1        192  Patient ID
sex        606      2   1.389439        1          2  Sex
bdate      606    192  -7784.267   -19533       4469  Date of birth
begdate    606    190   11390.11     9133      13514  Date of observation start
died       192      2   .2760417        0          1  Died
ddate      118     53   13696.07     9595      16426  Date of death
enddate    606     54   15902.48     9595      16436  Date of death/censoring
begage     606    192   52.49657  16.3258   83.35934  Age at observation start
endage     606    207   60.47696       20   92.18069  Age at death/censoring
_st        606      1          1        1          1
_d         606      2   .0874587        0          1
_t         606    207   60.47696       20   92.18069
_t0        606    207   57.03043  16.3258         90
agegr      606     16   56.27063       15         90  Age band
mrate      606     30   .0239183   .00027     .28071  Reference mortality rate
```

`strate` with the `smr()` option now calculates SMR; here we see it for each sex:

```
. strate sex, smr(mrate)

           failure _d:  died == 1
     analysis time _t:  endage
    enter on or after:  time begage
                   id:  patid

Estimated SMRs and lower/upper bounds of 95% confidence intervals
(606 records included in the analysis)

      sex    D      E      SMR    Lower    Upper

 1. male    34   36.37  0.9349   0.6680   1.3084
 2. female  19    9.50  1.9994   1.2753   3.1345
```

There are other commands that may be useful to estimate SMRs, such as `stptime` (see [ST] **stptime**) and `istdize` (see [R] **dstdize**). The `istdize` command requires considerable data preparation, so `strate` is much handier.

We can also use `poisson` to estimate SMR. As preparation, we must calculate the expected number of deaths and use that as the "exposure" instead of the time at risk. With the `irr` option, `poisson` does not display the constant, which is the estimate of interest, but we can obtain it with `lincom` after `poisson`.

```
. generate pyrs = _t - _t0

. label variable pyrs "Time at risk"

. replace died = _d
(414 real changes made)

. generate ediea = pyrs*mrate
```

```
. label variable edied "Expected deaths"
. poisson died if sex==2, exposure(edied) nolog
Poisson regression                          Number of obs  =        236
                                            LR chi2(0)     =       0.00
                                            Prob > chi2    =          .
Log likelihood = -77.492235                 Pseudo R2      =     0.0000
```

died	Coef.	Std. Err.	z	P>|z|	[95% Conf. Interval]
_cons	.6928325	.2294157	3.02	0.003	.2431859 1.142479
edied	(exposure)				

```
. lincom _cons, irr
 ( 1)  [died]_cons = 0
```

died	IRR	Std. Err.	z	P>|z|	[95% Conf. Interval]
(1)	1.999371	.4586871	3.02	0.003	1.275306 3.134529

For females, we found the same SMR as with strate. With poisson, we can also compare the SMRs for males and females; the SMR for females was significantly higher than that for males:

```
. poisson died sex, exposure(edied) irr nolog
Poisson regression                          Number of obs  =        606
                                            LR chi2(1)     =       6.44
                                            Prob > chi2    =     0.0112
Log likelihood = -225.56714                 Pseudo R2      =     0.0141
```

died	IRR	Std. Err.	z	P>|z|	[95% Conf. Interval]
sex	2.138617	.6125686	2.65	0.008	1.219893 3.749251
edied	(exposure)				

In the above example, we used Danish mortality from 1991 to 1995 as a reference, although the observations took place during 1985–2004. This was a bit quick and dirty, and if population mortality changed during the study period, we should use separate reference populations for different calendar periods. The necessary data manipulation corresponds to constructing a Lexis diagram; see Clayton and Hills (1993).

The reference mortality file dk1981-2004.dta includes the Danish age- and sex-specific mortality rates for the calendar periods 1981–1985, 1986–1990, 1991–1995, 1996–2000, and 2001–2004:

```
. use dk1981-2004.dta, clear

. summarize
    Variable |      Obs       Mean    Std. Dev.       Min        Max
    ---------+--------------------------------------------------------
        year |      210       1991    7.087964       1981       2001
         sex |      210        1.5    .5011947          1          2
       agegr |      210   45.28571    29.89958          0         95
       mrate |      210   .0496624    .0971473     .00008     .42985
```

To use this information, we should `stsplit` the patient data first by calendar time and next by age before merging it with the reference file. Splitting by calendar time requires that dates be transformed from days since 1 January 1960 to calendar years:

```
                         ———————— gen_oppatients3.do ————————
* gen_oppatients3.do

cd C:\docs\ishr2
use oppatients1.dta

* Transform dates to years since year 0.
  gen begyear = 1960 + begdate/365.25
  gen endyear = 1960 + enddate/365.25
  gen byear = 1960 + bdate/365.25

* stset with calendar time as time axis
  stset endyear, enter(time begyear) failure(died==1) id(patid)
* Split observations, one for each calendar time band
  stsplit timeband, at(1981 1986 1991 1996 2001 2006)
* recalculate age at start and end for each timeband
  replace begage = _t0 - byear
  replace endage = _t - byear

* stset with age as time axis
  stset endage, enter(time begage) failure(died==1) id(patid)
* Split observations once more, one for each age band
  stsplit agegr, at(0 1 5(5)100)

* Before merge with the reference file, variable names must match.
  rename timeband year
  sort year sex agegr
  merge year sex agegr using dk1981-2004.dta

* Now calculate expected number of deaths
  gen pyrs = _t - _t0
  gen edied = pyrs*mrate

save oppatients3.dta, replace
```

After we run merge by calendar time, sex, and age with the reference mortality file, we can estimate SMR, as before, by using strate or poisson:

```
. use oppatients3.dta
(Long term mortality after operation)

. strate sex, smr(mrate)

        failure _d:  died == 1
  analysis time _t:  endage
  enter on or after:  time begage
              id:  patid

Estimated SMRs and lower/upper bounds of 95% confidence intervals
(982 records included in the analysis)

        sex    D      E      SMR    Lower    Upper

   1. male    34  33.58  1.0124  0.7234   1.4168
   2. female  19   8.83  2.1515  1.3723   3.3730
```

Direct standardization

In direct standardization, the information in the age strata is weighted by the age distribution in a real or hypothetical population. We might, for example, see a curve of incidence development, adjusted to U.S. 1960 population, or a table of cancer incidence, adjusted to some European or world standard population.

You can download public-domain data on various standard populations from the U.S. National Cancer Institute's site: http://seer.cancer.gov/stdpopulations/. From these data, and from information at http://www.who.int/whosis/indicators/2007MortAgeStandardized/en/, I created a Stata dataset, stdpops.dta, with 12 different standard populations; it can be downloaded from this book's web site.

```
. use stdpops.dta

. tab1 standard

-> tabulation of standard
           standard |  Freq.    Percent     Cum.

      1. 2000 U.S. |    19      8.33       8.33
      2. 1940 U.S. |    19      8.33      16.67
      3. 1950 U.S. |    19      8.33      25.00
      4. 1960 U.S. |    19      8.33      33.33
      5. 1970 U.S. |    19      8.33      41.67
      6. 1980 U.S. |    19      8.33      50.00
      7. 1990 U.S. |    19      8.33      58.33
   8. 1991 Canadian |   19      8.33      66.67
   9. 1996 Canadian |   19      8.33      75.00
      10. European |    19      8.33      83.33
   11. World (Segi) |    19      8.33      91.67
    12. World (WHO) |    19      8.33     100.00

            Total |   228    100.00
```

To see the contents of the European standard, type

```
. list if standard==10, separator(0)
```

	standard	age	pop
172.	10. European	0. 0	16000
173.	10. European	1. 1-4	64000
174.	10. European	5. 5-9	70000
175.	10. European	10. 10-14	70000
176.	10. European	15. 15-19	70000
177.	10. European	20. 20-24	70000
178.	10. European	25. 25-29	70000
179.	10. European	30. 30-34	70000
180.	10. European	35. 35-39	70000
181.	10. European	40. 40-44	70000
182.	10. European	45. 45-49	70000
183.	10. European	50. 50-54	70000
184.	10. European	55. 55-59	60000
185.	10. European	60. 60-64	50000
186.	10. European	65. 65-69	40000
187.	10. European	70. 70-74	30000
188.	10. European	75. 75-79	20000
189.	10. European	80. 80-84	10000
190.	10. European	85. 85+	10000

dk1975-2004.dta contains mortality data for Danish males from 7 selected years:

```
. use dk1975-2004.dta
```

```
. summarize
```

Variable	Obs	Mean	Std. Dev.	Min	Max
age	133	40.31579	26.9973	0	85
year	133	1989.857	9.826636	1975	2004
deaths	133	1554.128	1802.25	20	5742
pop	133	135080.1	60133.45	16569	217770

The age distribution changed over the years, so to obtain comparable figures, we perform a direct standardization to the European standard population. First, we create the European standard population file from stdpops.dta:

```
——————————— gen_std_europe.do ———————————
* gen_std_europe.do

cd C:\docs\ishr2
use stdpops.dta
keep if standard==10
save std_europe.dta
```

The key variables age and pop have the same name in the dataset and the standard population file, and we can use dstdize:

```
. use dk1975-2004.dta

. dstdize deaths pop age, by(year) using(std_europe.dta)
```

-> year= 1975

Stratum	Pop.	Cases	Unadjusted Pop. Dist.	Stratum Rate[s]	Std. Pop. Dst[P]	s*P
0	35625	435	0.014	0.0122	0.016	0.0002
1	149186	101	0.060	0.0007	0.064	0.0000
5	202945	95	0.081	0.0005	0.070	0.0000
10	198652	83	0.079	0.0004	0.070	0.0000
15	190365	169	0.076	0.0009	0.070	0.0001
20	193301	234	0.077	0.0012	0.070	0.0001
25	217770	244	0.087	0.0011	0.070	0.0001
30	186095	216	0.074	0.0012	0.070	0.0001
35	151010	281	0.060	0.0019	0.070	0.0001
40	138301	413	0.055	0.0030	0.070	0.0002
45	139908	638	0.056	0.0046	0.070	0.0003
50	148380	1225	0.059	0.0083	0.070	0.0006
55	133749	1710	0.053	0.0128	0.060	0.0008
60	130096	2665	0.052	0.0205	0.050	0.0010
65	109128	3642	0.044	0.0334	0.040	0.0013
70	80260	4249	0.032	0.0529	0.030	0.0016
75	53210	4270	0.021	0.0802	0.020	0.0016
80	29667	3542	0.012	0.1194	0.010	0.0012
85	16569	3556	0.007	0.2146	0.010	0.0021

```
Totals:    2504217    27768      Adjusted Cases:   28806.6
                                    Crude Rate:     0.0111
                                 Adjusted Rate:     0.0115
                    95% Conf. Interval: [0.0114, 0.0116]
```

(output omitted)

Summary of Study Populations:

year	N	Crude	Adj_Rate	Confidence Interval	
1975	2504217	0.011088	0.011503	[0.011372,	0.011635]
1980	2529070	0.011938	0.011817	[0.011687,	0.011947]
1985	2517078	0.012130	0.011482	[0.011356,	0.011608]
1990	2530581	0.012317	0.011196	[0.011074,	0.011318]
1995	2573308	0.012151	0.010854	[0.010737,	0.010971]
2000	2634126	0.010733	0.009411	[0.009304,	0.009518]
2004	2677274	0.010271	0.008656	[0.008556,	0.008756]

The crude rates did not change much over the 30 years, but the adjusted rates did. Comparing the crude rates is misleading because of confounding by the changing age structure. However, the standard population is a choice, and with different weights, the results would have been different — although hardly dramatically so.

The standard populations in stdpops.dta are in 5-year age groups, but we might want to use coarser age strata:

```
——————————————————— gen_stdUS1990B.do ———————————
* gen_stdUS1990B.do

cd C:\docs\ishr2
use stdpops.dta
keep if standard==7
recode age (0 1=0 "0-4")(5 10=5 "5-14")(15/30=15 "15-34")     ///
    (35/50=35 "35-54") (55/70=55 "55-74")(75/max=75 "75+"),    ///
    generate(age2)
collapse (sum) pop, by(age2)
numlabel, add
rename age2 age

save stdUS1990B.dta
```

```
. list, separator(0)
```

	age	pop
1.	0. 0-4	73799
2.	5. 5-14	141584
3.	15. 15-34	321459
4.	35. 35-54	252512
5.	55. 55-74	157832
6.	75. 75+	52814

The name and coding of the age variable must be the same in your dataset and the standard population file; otherwise, `dstdize` will not work.

14.7   Some advanced issues

This section discusses some advanced issues that may or may not be important to you. If they are, you can read more in the *Survival Analysis and Epidemiological Tables Reference Manual* or in Cleves et al. (2008). Among topics not described in this book are parametric regression models (see [ST] **streg**) and random-effects models (see [ST] **stcox**).

Time-dependent covariates

In the analysis in section 14.3, we handled age as a time-dependent covariate: as time goes, age changes in a perfectly predictable way, and by letting age be the time axis, we could obtain an age-adjusted hazard ratio.

Also, imagine an event happening at some time during follow-up; the event could affect future risk, but hardly past risk. [ST] **stset** and [ST] **stcox** use the example of heart transplants in patients with serious heart disease. In principle, the solution is to split one observation in two: one censored at the time of a heart transplant and the other starting at the time of the heart transplant and ending with censoring or death. You can do this by using `stsplit`.

[ST] **stcox** also describes how to handle continuous time-dependent covariates.

Stratified regression

A stratified analysis is relevant when we have designed a matched cohort study, such as one matching one or more unexposed persons to each exposed person by age and sex. Assuming that the persons in a matched set share baseline risk (apart from the exposure), we specify the `strata()` option. Here the variable `setid` identifies the matched sets:

```
. stcox x1 x2, strata(setid)
```

The principle is much the same as in conditional logistic regression, where the `group()` option identifies the matched sets; see section 13.4.

Multiple-failure data

In a standard survival analysis, we look at one event per person, and when the event has happened, it's over; death is the obvious example. Multiple events, such as hospital admissions, are often analyzed with the same model using the time to first admission only, but doing that leaves a lot of useful information unused. On the other hand, multiple admissions cannot be treated as independent events.

The solution described in [ST] **stcox** involves specifying the observations for each person as a cluster by the `vce(cluster clustvar)` option. (The `vce(robust)` option has the same effect, provided that the `stset` command included the `id()` option.) This example is similar to the repeated-observations problem described in section 13.4.

```
. stcox x1 x2, vce(cluster id)
```

Competing events

How do we handle deaths from other causes (competing events or risks) if we study mortality from a specific disease? A classical way to handle this is to censor observations at the time of death from any other cause, to estimate the cumulative mortality from this cause if there had been no other causes of death. This situation is counterfactual, but well defined.

The term *cumulative incidence* is used in (at least) two different meanings. The first type is the classical 1 − KM (the Kaplan–Meier survival estimate with deaths from other causes being censored). A second type is an estimate obtained by a modification ensuring that the sum of cause-specific cumulative mortality estimates equals the total cumulative mortality. In the presence of competing risks, the latter cause-specific cumulative incidence becomes lower than the classical estimate; see Farley, Ali, and Slaymaker (2001).

(Continued on next page)

What is "right" depends on the question asked. If you, from the manufacturer's point of view, study the durability (or time to failure) of some kind of prosthesis, death of a patient from unrelated causes obviously prevents you from learning more about this patient's prosthesis, and the classical method of censoring at the time of death answers the question. However, from the patient's perspective, it is relevant to take the risk of dying from something unrelated into consideration. Here the question may be whether the prosthesis will fail before the patient dies from something else.

The official Stata `st` commands are designed to handle competing events the classical way. `stcompet` estimates the second type of cumulative incidence; see Coviello and Boggess (2004). However, there is no test like a log-rank test available, nor is there any regression model available. `stcompet` is not an official Stata command, but you can find and download it by typing

```
. findit stcompet
```

15 Measurement and diagnosis

15.1 Reproducibility of measurements

Categorical measurements: The kappa statistic

Two radiologists independently classified 85 mammograms (Altman 1990). The results are recorded in rate2.dta. I used numlabel to add codes to the value labels, and I requested a cross table:

```
. webuse rate2.dta
(Altman p. 403)

. numlabel, add

. tab2 rada radb

-> tabulation of rada by radb

Radiologis |
      t A's |           Radiologist B's assessment
 assessment | 1. Normal  2. benign  3. suspec  4. cancer |     Total
------------+--------------------------------------------+----------
  1. Normal |        21         12          0          0 |        33
  2. benign |         4         17          1          0 |        22
 3. suspect |         3          9         15          2 |        29
  4. cancer |         0          0          0          1 |         1
------------+--------------------------------------------+----------
      Total |        28         38         16          3 |        85
```

Among the 85 cases, we find agreement between the two raters in $21 + 17 + 15 + 1 = 54$ cases (63.5%). However, we would expect agreement by pure chance in 30.8% of the cases (we calculate the expected cell values from the marginal distributions). The kappa statistic expresses the amount of agreement beyond the chance expectation. It has the flavor of a correlation coefficient, with 1 indicating perfect agreement and 0, no more than chance agreement. It has been suggested that we interpret kappa values above 0.80 as "almost perfect" and kappa values above 0.60 as "good", but it may be problematic to assign such labels mechanically to a statistic without regard to the problem at hand.

The kap command (see [R] **kappa**) requires that the data structure be wide, i.e., that the two ratings to be compared are in the same observation.

```
. kap rada radb

             |  Expected
   Agreement | Agreement     Kappa   Std. Err.        Z     Prob>Z
-------------+------------------------------------------------------
      63.53% |    30.82%    0.4728      0.0694      6.81     0.0000
```

259

With an ordinal scale, as in the above example, we see that some disagreements are larger than others, and we may want to let small disagreements (benign versus suspect) have less weight than large disagreements (normal versus cancer). The `wgt(w)` option automatically weights the agreements according to distance:

```
. kap rada radb, wgt(w)
Ratings weighted by:
    1.0000    0.6667    0.3333    0.0000
    0.6667    1.0000    0.6667    0.3333
    0.3333    0.6667    1.0000    0.6667
    0.0000    0.3333    0.6667    1.0000

                  Expected
 Agreement       Agreement      Kappa     Std. Err.            Z      Prob>Z

   86.67%          69.11%      0.5684        0.0788         7.22      0.0000
```

You can control distance weights, and it is possible to express the agreement between several raters.

Continuous measurements: Assessing measurement variation

Generally accepted principles for assessing and comparing measurements have been described by Bland and Altman (1986); for a more recent and instructive text, see Bland and Altman (2003). You can find textbook descriptions in Bland (2000) and Kirkwood and Sterne (2003).

The dataset `anklebp1.dta` contains data for 107 patients with suspected arterial insufficiency in the legs (the dataset includes one leg per patient). Ankle blood pressure was measured twice at the dorsal pedal artery (adp1, adp2) and twice at the posterior tibial artery (atp1, atp2).

```
. cd C:\docs\ishr2
c:\docs\ishr2

. use anklebp1.dta
(Ankle blood pressure data)

. codebook, compact

Variable    Obs Unique      Mean   Min   Max   Label

id          107    107   97.26168     1   194   Patient id
adp1        107     26    116.729    30   195   a.dorsalis pedis (1)
adp2        107     30   117.3364    30   200   a.dorsalis pedis (2)
atp1        107     29   117.9907    30   190   a.tibialis posterior (1)
atp2        107     30   118.3925    30   190   a.tibialis posterior (2)
```

We want to assess the variation of measurement at each site and to compare results from the two sites. Correlation coefficients give us a hint — but not more:

```
. correlate adp1-atp2
(obs=107)
                 adp1      adp2      atp1      atp2
        adp1   1.0000
        adp2   0.9800    1.0000
        atp1   0.9276    0.9298    1.0000
        atp2   0.9291    0.9329    0.9881    1.0000
```

Within each site, the correlation coefficients are high (0.98–0.99), but between sites they are more modest (0.93). A matrix graph gives a nice visual display (see figure 15.1):

```
. graph matrix adp1-atp2, half ysize(3) xsize(3.1)
```

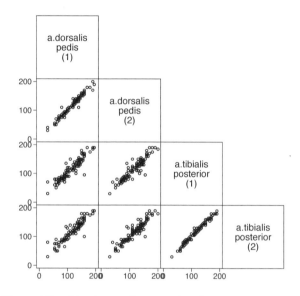

Figure 15.1. Matrix graph comparing four measurements

The matrix graph confirms the impression from the correlation coefficients: there is little variation between same-site measurements and somewhat more variation between different-site measurements. Looking at the codebook output above, we can see that the differences between same-site means are small. We now want to express the measurement variation for each site as a variance or standard deviation; to do this, we must reshape the data to long format:

(Continued on next page)

```
─────────────────────── gen_anklebp2.do ───────────────────────
* gen_anklebp2.do

cd C:\docs\ishr2
use anklebp1.dta
reshape long atp adp, i(id) j(meas)

label data "Ankle blood pressure data; long format"
save anklebp2.dta
```

After we run `reshape` (see section 9.6), the data structure is

```
. list in 1/6, sepby(id)
```

	id	meas	adp	atp
1.	1	1	105	105
2.	1	2	110	105
3.	2	1	110	110
4.	2	2	110	110
5.	4	1	140	150
6.	4	2	130	160

A oneway analysis of variance will show us the within-individual variation of measurements on the dorsal pedal artery:

```
. oneway adp id
```

	Analysis of Variance				
Source	SS	df	MS	F	Prob > F
Between groups	271178.271	106	2558.28558	99.09	0.0000
Within groups	2762.5	107	25.817757		
Total	273940.771	213	1286.10691		

```
Bartlett's test for equal variances:  chi2(67) =  33.2114  Prob>chi2 = 1.000

note: Bartlett's test performed on cells with positive variance:
      39 multiple-observation cells not used
```

The within-groups mean square, MS, is the intraindividual variance (25.8), and its square root is the intraindividual variation expressed as standard deviation (5.1 mmHg). We can thus estimate, from the normal distribution, that in about 68% of the observations the deviation from the individual mean was within 5.1 mmHg, and in 95% of the observations, within 10 mmHg. For the atp measurements, the intraindividual variation (standard deviation) was 3.9 mmHg.

loneway (see [R] **loneway**) gives some supplementary information:

```
. loneway adp id
                    One-way Analysis of Variance for adp:
                                                Number of obs =        214
                                                R-squared =     0.9899

        Source            SS        df       MS           F      Prob > F

    Between id       271178.27      106    2558.2856      99.09    0.0000
    Within id           2762.5      107    25.817757

    Total            273940.77      213    1286.1069

            Intraclass       Asy.
            correlation      S.E.          [95% Conf. Interval]

             0.98002        0.00383        0.97250       0.98753

        Estimated SD of id effect                 35.58418
        Estimated SD within id                     5.081118
        Est. reliability of a id mean              0.98991
                (evaluated at n=2.00)
```

Here we find the estimated variance and standard deviation within id. The intraclass correlation coefficient has the same problems of interpretation as any other correlation coefficient: it depends on the variation both within and between subjects, and when assessing measurement variation we are interested in the within-subjects variation only. The intraclass correlation coefficient and a weighted kappa coefficient can be interpreted much the same way.

15.2 Comparing methods of measurement

The intraindividual variation of the adp and atp measurements was small, so we use the mean of two measurements for comparison of results from the two sites. We generate a modified dataset, anklebp3.dta, including some derived variables:

```
———————————————— gen_anklebp3.do ————————————————
* gen_anklebp3.do

cd C:\docs\ishr2
use anklebp1.dta

generate adpmean=(adp1+adp2)/2
generate atpmean=(atp1+atp2)/2
generate ankledif=adpmean-atpmean
generate anklemean=(adpmean+atpmean)/2

save anklebp3.dta
```

We examine the correlation between the mean from each site. A correlation coefficient of 0.94 looks satisfactory, but beware: a correlation coefficient does not tell whether the results from the two sites are identical. If the adp measurements were consistently half the atp measurements, we would get a high correlation coefficient anyway:

```
. use anklebp3.dta
(Ankle blood pressure data)

. correlate adpmean atpmean
(obs=107)

             │ adpmean  atpmean
 ────────────┼──────────────────
     adpmean │  1.0000
     atpmean │  0.9374   1.0000
```

The most important tool is graphical, and we draw a simple scatterplot with an identity line (figure 15.2). We want a square scatterplot, hence the aspectratio(1) option:

```
────────────────────── gph_fig15_2.do ──────────────────────
* gph_fig15_2.do

cd C:\docs\ishr2
use anklebp3.dta
set scheme lean1

twoway                                      ///
  (scatter adpmean atpmean)                 ///
  (function y=x, range(0 200) lpattern(l))  ///
  ,                                         ///
  legend(off)                               ///
  xtitle(atp) ytitle(adp)                   ///
  ysize(2.2) xsize(3) aspectratio(1) scale(1.4)
```

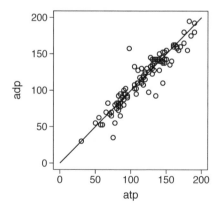

Figure 15.2. Scatterplot with identity line

The line is the identity line (adp = atp), not a regression line. Even in the absence of bias, a regression line would have a slope of less than one because of regression toward the mean. We can compare means with a paired t test and become satisfied:

```
. ttest adpmean==atpmean

Paired t test
```

Variable	Obs	Mean	Std. Err.	Std. Dev.	[95% Conf. Interval]	
adpmean	107	117.0327	3.457543	35.76511	110.1778	123.8876
atpmean	107	118.1916	3.400341	35.1734	111.4501	124.9331
diff	107	-1.158879	1.215053	12.5686	-3.567839	1.250082

```
        mean(diff) = mean(adpmean - atpmean)                      t =  -0.9538
    Ho: mean(diff) = 0                         degrees of freedom =      106

    Ha: mean(diff) < 0            Ha: mean(diff) != 0            Ha: mean(diff) > 0
    Pr(T < t) = 0.1712         Pr(|T| > |t|) = 0.3424            Pr(T > t) = 0.8288
```

In a Bland–Altman plot, the difference between two measurements is plotted against their mean. The procedure does not exist in official Stata, but let's see if there are any user-written commands by typing

```
. findit bland altman
```

This command leads to the following information:

```
STB-55  sbe33 . . . . Comparing several methods of measuring the same quantity
        (help baplot, bagroup, bamat, sdpair if installed) . . . . . P. Seed
        5/00     pp.2--9; STB Reprints Vol 10, pp.73--82
        commands implementing the Bland-Altman approach to comparing
        two or more measurement methods;  also alternative command to
        sdtest based on Pitman's method giving confidence intervals
        for variance ratios of paired data
```

After clicking on sbe33, installing the package, and reading the help file, we can examine the result:

```
. baplot adpmean atpmean

Bland-Altman comparison of adpmean and atpmean
Limits of agreement (Reference Range for difference): -26.296 to 23.978
Mean difference: -1.159 (CI -3.568 to  1.250)
Range : 30.000 to 191.250
Pitman's Test of difference in variance: r =  0.048, n = 107, p = 0.625
```

The mean difference gives the same result as the paired t test above. It was not significant: -1.16 mmHg (95% CI: -3.57, 1.25). The *limits of agreement* describe a 95% reference range or prediction interval $(-26.3, 24.0)$ for the difference between the two measurements. If we assume a normal distribution, we expect 95% of the observed differences to lie within this interval. We also get a graph in the old Stata style (not shown), but with the output information, it is not too difficult to create one using modern graphics (figure 15.3):

```
──────── gph_fig15_3.do ────────
* gph_fig15_3.do

cd C:\docs\ishr2
use anklebp3.dta

twoway                                   ///
  (scatter ankledif anklemean)           ///
  ,                                       ///
  ytitle("Difference")                    ///
  xtitle("Average")                       ///
  ylabel(-50(25)50)                       ///
  yline(-1.159, lpattern(1))              ///
  yline(-26.296 23.978, lpattern(dash))   ///
  ysize(2.2) xsize(3.1) scale(1.4)
```

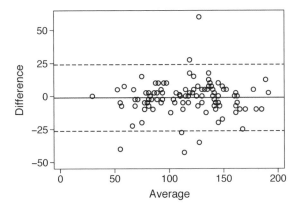

Figure 15.3. Bland–Altman plot of difference versus average of two measurements

The Bland–Altman plot can be used to examine whether the measurement differences depend on the blood pressure level (similarly to examining a residual plot to assess heteroskedasticity; section 13.1). This seems not to be the case. The mean difference is close to 0, so there is no systematic difference in results from the two sites. In 95% of paired observations, the difference was within 25 mmHg, and the remaining question is whether this finding is satisfactory from a clinical point of view.

The analysis performed does not permit us to determine which artery gives the most valid results, but comparing the intraindividual variations might give a clue. sdpair (downloaded with the package for Bland–Altman analysis) lets us compare the standard deviations between differences (dadp and datp):

```
. use anklebp1.dta
(Ankle blood pressure data)

. generate dadp = adp1-adp2

. generate datp = atp1-atp2

. sdpair datp dadp

Pitman's variance ratio test between datp and dadp:

Ratio of Standard deviations = 0.7592
95% Confidence Interval 0.6265 to 0.9200
t = -2.862, df = 105, p =  0.005
```

Pitman's variance-ratio test shows that the intraindividual variation is significantly smaller for atp than for adp, and we can interpret this to mean that atp is the most precise measurement. Whether the differences are clinically important is another question, and we would like to compare with a clinically meaningful external criterion, a "gold standard". This question will be addressed in more detail in the following section.

15.3   Using tests for diagnosis

If we have a "gold standard", i.e., a chosen criterion of truth, we can estimate the agreement between a test and the truth it is meant to measure. I recommend reading Sackett et al. (1991). A statistically more advanced text is given by Pepe (2003).

The data used in this section are partly constructed, and they should not be used as evidence when considering diagnosis of renal artery stenosis. The ras.dta dataset is a modified version of the data used by Habbema et al. (2002). These data consist of 437 patients who were suspected of renal artery stenosis and who had angiography performed, and the result of the angiography was considered the criterion of truth. However, angiography is an invasive procedure, carrying some risk to the patient, and the question was whether less-risky and less-expensive procedures could be used for diagnostic purposes and reduce the number of patients exposed to angiography. The dataset includes the following variables:

```
. use ras.dta
(Diagnosis of renal artery stenosis)

. codebook, compact

Variable   Obs Unique     Mean  Min  Max  Label

patid      437    437      219    1  437  Patient ID
stenosis   437      2  .228833    0    1  Stenosis at angiography
renogram   437      2 .2379863    0    1  Abnormal renography
crea       437    102 93.12815   51  189  S-creatinine, micro-mol/L
creagrp    437     10 88.09382   51  151  S-creatinine, grouped
```

Dichotomous tests

The renogram is a noninvasive imaging test. This test can be positive, indicating possible renal ischemia, or negative (things are, no doubt, more complicated than that). First, let's look at a cross table between angiography and renography results:

```
. tab2 renogram stenosis, col
-> tabulation of renogram by stenosis
```

Key
frequency *column percentage*

Abnormal renography	Stenosis at angiography 0. no 1. yes	Total
0. no	304 29 90.21 29.00	333 76.20
1. yes	33 71 9.79 71.00	104 23.80
Total	337 100 100.00 100.00	437 100.00

Among the 437 patients, 100 (23%) had stenosis at angiography. Among those with stenosis, 71% had an abnormal renography, while among other patients, it was 10%.

To estimate the sensitivity and specificity of renography in diagnosing renal artery stenosis, we can use ci with the binomial option (see section 10.5 and [R] **ci**):

```
. bysort stenosis: ci renogram, binomial
```

```
-> stenosis = 0. no
```

Variable	Obs	Mean	Std. Err.	— Binomial Exact — [95% Conf. Interval]
renogram	337	.0979228	.0161901	.068368 .134768

```
-> stenosis = 1. yes
```

Variable	Obs	Mean	Std. Err.	— Binomial Exact — [95% Conf. Interval]
renogram	100	.71	.0453762	.610734 .7964258

The sensitivity is estimated to be 0.71 (95% CI: 0.61, 0.80) and the specificity to be $1 - 0.098 = 0.90$ (95% CI: 0.87, 0.93). In the same manner, we could estimate the positive and negative predictive values in this patient population by using

```
. by renogram, sort: ci stenosis, binomial
```

Official Stata has no commands with the specific purpose to estimate sensitivity, specificity, and predictive values, but with

```
. findit sensitivity specificity
```

we locate

```
SJ-4-4  sbe36_2 . . . . . . . . . . . . . . . . . . Software update for diagt
        (help diagt if installed) . . . . . . . . . P. T. Seed and A. Tobias
        Q4/04   SJ 4(4):490
        new options added to diagt
```

Information on this procedure was published in the *Stata Journal*, Volume 4, Number 4. Click on the link sbe36_2, install diagt, and then read the help file. To estimate the parameters of interest, type

```
. diagt stenosis renogram
```

Stenosis at angiograph y	Abnormal renography Pos.	Neg.	Total
Abnormal	71	29	100
Normal	33	304	337
Total	104	333	437

True abnormal diagnosis defined as stenosis = 1 (labelled 1. yes)

			[95% Confidence Interval]	
Prevalence	Pr(A)	23%	19%	27.1%
Sensitivity	Pr(+|A)	71%	61.1%	79.6%
Specificity	Pr(-|N)	90.2%	86.5%	93.2%
ROC area	(Sens. + Spec.)/2	.806	.759	.853
Likelihood ratio (+)	Pr(+|A)/Pr(+|N)	7.25	5.12	10.3
Likelihood ratio (-)	Pr(-|A)/Pr(-|N)	.321	.236	.438
Odds ratio	LR(+)/LR(-)	22.6	12.9	39.5
Positive predictive value	Pr(A|+)	68.3%	58.4%	77.1%
Negative predictive value	Pr(N|-)	91.3%	87.7%	94.1%

The table reports sensitivity and specificity and the receiver operating characteristic (ROC) area. The (rather unusual) ROC curve can be shown with

```
. roctab stenosis renogram, graph
```

An ROC area of 1 means perfect agreement, and an area of 0.5 means that there is no more than random agreement. Sensitivity and specificity are combined in likelihood ratios for positive and negative test results, and the ratio between these is the odds ratio from the 2×2 table.

The positive and negative predictive value estimates are valid for the actual study population and for similar patient populations with the same prior probability of disease (disease prevalence 23%). We may now ask, how would the test perform in a population with a different prior risk of disease, such as 10%? This can be examined by including the prev() option in the diagt command:

```
. diagt stenosis renogram, prev(10%)
```

(output omitted)

			[95% Confidence Interval]		
Prevalence	Pr(A)	10%	── (given) ──		
Sensitivity	Pr(+|A)	71%	61.1%	79.6%	
Specificity	Pr(-|N)	90.2%	86.5%	93.2%	
ROC area	(Sens. + Spec.)/2	.806	.759	.853	
Likelihood ratio (+)	Pr(+|A)/Pr(+|N)	7.25	5.12	10.3	
Likelihood ratio (-)	Pr(-|A)/Pr(-|N)	.321	.236	.438	
Odds ratio	LR(+)/LR(-)	22.6	12.9	39.5	
Positive predictive value	Pr(A|+)	44.6%	36.3%	53.3%	(lr)
Negative predictive value	Pr(N|-)	96.6%	95.4%	97.4%	(lr)
Pre-test odds	prev/(1-prev)	.111	── (given) ──		
Post-test odds (+)	Pr(A|+)/(1-Pr(A|+))	.806	.569	1.14	(lr)
Post-test odds (-)	Pr(A|-)/(1-Pr(A|-))	.0357	.0486	.0262	(lr)

```
(lr) Values and confidence intervals are based on likelihood
     ratios, assuming that the prevalence is known exactly.
```

As expected, the positive predictive value decreased and the negative predictive value increased when applying the test in a population with lower prior risk of disease. The calculations depend on sensitivity and specificity being the same in different patient populations, and that assumption may be questioned; see, e.g., Sackett and Haynes (2002).

Continuous tests

With continuous tests, e.g., biochemical concentrations, sensitivity and specificity can be estimated for a chosen cutpoint. Typically there is a trade-off so that moving the cutpoint to increase sensitivity reduces specificity and vice versa. ROC analysis can give an overall estimate of the discriminatory power of a continuous test. See [R] **roc** for a description of the family of commands useful for ROC analysis.

The main parameter of interest is the area under the curve. For a perfect test, the area is 1; for a test with no association between test result and disease status, the area is 0.5. Using crea (serum creatinine) as the test, roctab calculates the area under the curve; it is 0.70 (95% CI: 0.64, 0.76). roctab with the graph option displays the ROC curve (figure 15.4); see the full command (gph_fig15_4.do) at this book's web site.

```
. roctab stenosis crea, summary graph
```

	ROC		─Asymptotic Normal─	
Obs	Area	Std. Err.	[95% Conf. Interval]	
437	0.7009	0.0309	0.64034	0.76153

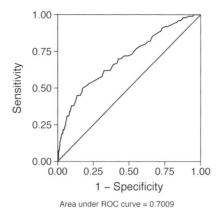

Figure 15.4. ROC curve: Serum creatinine as predictor of renal artery stenosis

The ROC curve does not display test values, but the `detail` option creates a table. To avoid a huge table, I used the grouped variable `creagrp`. We cannot, however, determine the optimal cutpoint without considering health and cost consequences of false negative and false positive test results. The value labels are a bit misleading in the table, so I detach them from `creagrp` first:

```
. label values creagrp
. roctab stenosis creagrp, detail
```
Detailed report of Sensitivity and Specificity

Cutpoint	Sensitivity	Specificity	Correctly Classified	LR+	LR-
(>= 51)	100.00%	0.00%	22.88%	1.0000	
(>= 61)	99.00%	5.64%	27.00%	1.0492	0.1774
(>= 71)	95.00%	16.32%	34.32%	1.1353	0.3064
(>= 81)	82.00%	36.20%	46.68%	1.2853	0.4972
(>= 91)	70.00%	57.27%	60.18%	1.6382	0.5238
(>= 101)	53.00%	78.34%	72.54%	2.4467	0.6000
(>= 111)	38.00%	90.50%	78.49%	4.0019	0.6850
(>= 121)	31.00%	93.47%	79.18%	4.7486	0.7382
(>= 131)	22.00%	96.14%	79.18%	5.7031	0.8113
(>= 151)	11.00%	98.52%	78.49%	7.4140	0.9034
(> 151)	0.00%	100.00%	77.12%		1.0000

Obs	ROC Area	Std. Err.	—Asymptotic Normal— [95% Conf. Interval]	
437	0.7028	0.0309	0.64219	0.76333

The `roccomp` command lets us compare two or more tests or compare subgroups of observations. Here we compare the creatinine–stenosis association among patients with and without abnormal renogram (see figure 15.5):

```
. roccomp stenosis crea, by(renogram) summary graph
```

		ROC		—Asymptotic Normal—	
renogram	Obs	Area	Std. Err.	[95% Conf. Interval]	
0	333	0.5698	0.0473	0.47709	0.66254
1	104	0.6921	0.0588	0.57683	0.80730

```
Ho: area(0) = area(1)
    chi2(1) =    2.62        Prob>chi2 =   0.1053
```

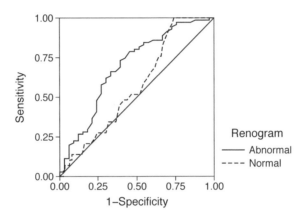

Figure 15.5. ROC curves for creatinine among patients with abnormal and normal renogram

You can find the full graph command (`gph_fig15_5.do`) at this book's web site.

It seems from the table and the graph that there was almost no association between creatinine level and stenosis among patients with a normal renogram, while there was a significant association among patients with an abnormal renogram. However, the areas under the curve were not significantly different ($Pr = 0.11$). In both groups, the area under the curve was smaller than in the overall analysis (figure 15.4). Serum creatinine and renography results are not independent, and with knowledge of the renography result, the discriminatory power of serum creatinine diminishes.

15.4 Combining test results

In section 15.3, we saw that both the renogram result and the serum-creatinine level contributed to the prediction of stenosis. The likelihood ratio for an abnormal renogram was 7.25, and the likelihood ratio for serum creatinine ≥ 111 μmol/L was 4.00, and we might want to combine the information. The prior odds of stenosis were $100/337 = 0.297$, and the odds of stenosis in a patient with an abnormal renogram and serum creatinine ≥ 111 μmol/L are $0.297 \times 7.25 \times 4.00 = 8.613$. The corresponding probability is $8.613/9.613 = 0.90$.

This calculation ignores the fact that the renography result and serum creatinine are not independent. To allow for dependence, perform a logistic regression:

```
. use ras.dta
(Diagnosis of renal artery stenosis)

. logistic stenosis renogram crea
```

```
Logistic regression                              Number of obs   =        437
                                                 LR chi2(2)      =     152.91
                                                 Prob > chi2     =     0.0000
Log likelihood = -158.59076                      Pseudo R2       =     0.3253
```

stenosis	Odds Ratio	Std. Err.	z	P>|z|	[95% Conf. Interval]	
renogram	17.68998	5.228973	9.72	0.000	9.911079	31.57429
crea	1.017621	.005813	3.06	0.002	1.006291	1.029078

The `lroc` command after `logistic` draws an ROC curve and calculates the area under the curve (see figure 15.6):

```
. lroc

Logistic model for stenosis

number of observations =        437
area under ROC curve    =     0.8377
```

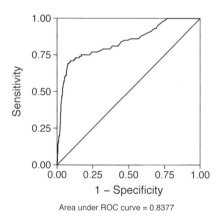

Figure 15.6. ROC curve utilizing the combined results from renography and serum creatinine

When we compare it with the areas found in section 15.3 for renography (0.806) and serum creatinine (0.701), the combination of tests has greater discriminatory power. However, `lroc` does not display the confidence interval for the area; to obtain that, we use `predict` after `logistic` and use the predicted probability (prob) as input to `roctab`. For information on `predict`, see section 13.1.

```
. predict prob if e(sample)
(option pr assumed; Pr(stenosis))

. roctab stenosis prob, summary
                         ROC                      —Asymptotic Normal—
              Obs        Area      Std. Err.      [95% Conf. Interval]

              437       0.8377       0.0252        0.78818      0.88713
```

An ROC curve does not show the actual test values, but we can use `adjust` after `logistic` (see section 13.2) to get the probability of disease with a given combination of test values. For patients with a serum creatinine of 70 μmol/L, the probability of stenosis with normal and abnormal renograms is estimated by typing

```
. quietly logistic stenosis renogram crea

. adjust crea=70, by(renogram) pr ci
```

```
       Dependent variable: stenosis      Command: logistic
       Covariate set to value: crea = 70


    Abnormal
    renograph
    y                    pr            lb            ub

       0. no         .061929      [.039741      .095274]
       1. yes        .538711      [.401669      .670141]

       Key:   pr        =   Probability
              [lb , ub] =   [95% Confidence Interval]
```

With one continuous and one categorical test, we can graph the predicted probability (prob) obtained by `predict` for any combination of test results. The data must be sorted by crea before graphing (see figure 15.7):

```
. sort crea

. twoway (line prob crea if renogram==1)(line prob crea if renogram==0)
```

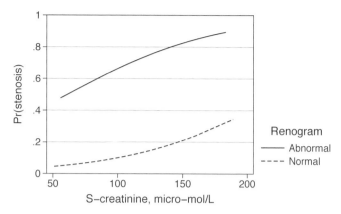

Figure 15.7. Predicted probability of stenosis, by renography and serum-creatinine results

If we — considering the benefits, risks, and costs associated with angiography — decide that angiography is indicated if the predicted probability of stenosis is at least 10%, the rule should be that angiography is offered to all patients with an abnormal renogram and to patients with serum creatinine > 100 μmol/L. This would lead to angiography being offered to 181 (41%) of the initially suspected patients, with a positive predictive value of 43% and a negative predictive value of 91%.

```
. generate p10 = prob>0.10 if prob<.
. diagt stenosis p10

   Stenosis |
         at |
  angiograph|           p10
          y |    Pos.       Neg. |     Total
  ----------+---------------------+----------
    Abnormal |     78         22 |       100
      Normal |    103        234 |       337
  ----------+---------------------+----------
       Total |    181        256 |       437

True abnormal diagnosis defined as stenosis = 1 (labelled 1. yes)
```

			[95% Confidence Interval]	
Prevalence	Pr(A)	23%	19%	27.1%
Sensitivity	Pr(+|A)	78%	68.6%	85.7%
Specificity	Pr(−|N)	69.4%	64.2%	74.3%
ROC area	(Sens. + Spec.)/2	.737	.69	.785
Likelihood ratio (+)	Pr(+|A)/Pr(+|N)	2.55	2.11	3.09
Likelihood ratio (−)	Pr(−|A)/Pr(−|N)	.317	.218	.461
Odds ratio	LR(+)/LR(−)	8.05	4.77	13.6
Positive predictive value	Pr(A|+)	43.1%	35.8%	50.6%
Negative predictive value	Pr(N|−)	91.4%	87.3%	94.5%

16 Miscellaneous

16.1 Random samples, simulations

Random-number functions

The fundamental random-number function in Stata is `uniform()` (no arguments, just empty parentheses). It creates pseudorandom numbers, uniformly distributed in the interval 0–1:

```
. generate y = uniform()
```

The term "pseudorandom" refers to the fact that no computer program can generate number sequences that are truly random, but you can generate number sequences that exhibit no predictable pattern.

The `uniform()` function can be combined with other functions and operators (see [D] **functions**) to obtain random numbers with a desired distribution:

```
. generate y = invnormal(uniform())
```
Normal distribution,
mean $= 0$, SD $= 1$

```
. generate y = 10 + 2*invnormal(uniform())
```
Normal distribution,
mean $= 10$, SD $= 2$

If you run the same command twice, it will yield different number sequences. If you need to reproduce the same series of "random" numbers, initialize the seed (a large integer used for the initial calculations), for example,

```
. set seed 654321
```

Random samples and randomization

You can use `sample` to select a random sample of your dataset (see [D] **sample**), for example,

```
. sample 10          Select an approximately 10% random sample
. sample 53, count   Select exactly 53 observations at random
```

You can assign observations randomly to two treatments by typing, for example,

```
. generate y = uniform()
. generate treat = 1
. replace treat = 0 if y<0.5
```

The same result can be obtained with one command. uniform()>0.5 evaluates to 1 if it is true; otherwise, it evaluates to 0:

```
. generate treat = uniform()>0.5
```

You can sort your observations in random sequence:

```
. generate treat = uniform()
. sort treat
```

Generating artificial datasets

You can use set obs to create empty observations. The following sequence creates a file with 10,000 observations, used to study the behavior of the difference (dif) between two measurements (x1, x2), given information about components of variance (sdwithin, sdbetw):

```
. clear
. set seed 654321
. set obs 10000
obs was 0, now 10000
. generate sdbetw = 20
. generate sdwithin = 10
. generate x0 = 50 + sdbetw * invnormal(uniform())
. generate x1 = x0 + sdwithin * invnormal(uniform())
. generate x2 = x0 + sdwithin * invnormal(uniform())
. generate dif = x2 - x1
. summarize
```

Variable	Obs	Mean	Std. Dev.	Min	Max
sdbetw	10000	20	0	20	20
sdwithin	10000	10	0	10	10
x0	10000	49.67348	20.20338	-22.72752	121.5295
x1	10000	49.52737	22.56641	-38.01537	146.0267
x2	10000	49.7786	22.66963	-29.34487	143.6227
dif	10000	.2512316	14.17881	-56.3431	51.27083

However, because sdbetw and sdwithin are constants, you do not need to create them as variables; it is more efficient to define them as scalars (see section 17.2), and part of the above commands could be

```
. ...
. scalar SDB = 20
. scalar SDW = 10
. generate x0 = 50 + SDB * invnormal(uniform())
. generate x1 = x0 + SDW * invnormal(uniform())
. generate x2 = x0 + SDW * invnormal(uniform())
. ...
```

Advanced simulations

With `simulate`, we can set up complex Monte Carlo simulations; see [R] **simulate**. You might also want to study [R] **bootstrap**, [R] **jackknife**, and [R] **permute** for more advanced topics.

16.2   Sample size and study power

Sample-size and study-power estimation are prestudy activities. What are the consequences of different decisions and assumptions for sample size and study power? The immediate command `sampsi` lets us calculate the required sample size or the power of a study; see [R] **sampsi**.

We must make the following decisions:

- The desired significance level (α); the default is 0.05 (two-sided)
- The minimum relevant contrast that you do not want to miss, expressed as study group means or proportions
- For sample-size estimation: the desired power ($1 - \beta$); the default is 0.90
- For power estimation: sample sizes

With comparison of means, you must also make an assumption: the assumed standard deviation in each sample.

Table 16.1 shows some short examples for the four main scenarios.

Table 16.1. Sample-size and power estimation examples

Comparison of	Sample-size estimation	Power estimation
Proportions	`sampsi 0.4 0.5`	`sampsi 0.4 0.5, n(60)`
Means	`sampsi 50 60, sd(8)`	`sampsi 50 60, sd(8) n(60)`

(Continued on next page)

Table 16.2 shows further options that are available.

Table 16.2. Further options for sample-size and power estimation

Situation	Options	Sample-size estimation Proportions	Means	Power estimation Proportions	Means
Significance level; default: 0.05	`alpha(0.01)`	+	+	+	+
Power; default: 0.90	`power(0.95)`	+	+		
Unequal sample sizes; ratio = n2/n1	`ratio(2)`	+	+		
Unequal sample sizes	`n1(40) n2(80)`			+	+
Unequal SDs	`sd1(6) sd2(9)`		+		+

Here is an example showing a sample-size estimation for a comparison of means with unequal SDs and unequal sample sizes:

```
. sampsi 50 60, sd1(14) sd2(10) ratio(2)
Estimated sample size for two-sample comparison of means

Test Ho: m1 = m2, where m1 is the mean in population 1
                    and m2 is the mean in population 2

Assumptions:

         alpha =   0.0500  (two-sided)
         power =   0.9000
            m1 =       50
            m2 =       60
           sd1 =       14
           sd2 =       10
         n2/n1 =     2.00

Estimated required sample sizes:
            n1 =       26
            n2 =       52
```

`sampsi` also handles trials with repeated measurements; see [R] **sampsi**. Rather than remembering the exact syntax, you may want to use the dialog:

```
. db sampsi
```

For incidence, mortality, and survival studies (see chapter 14), there are a couple of sample-size and power estimation commands; see [ST] **stpower**.

Here I show an example of `stpower logrank`, corresponding to a simple comparison of incidence in two groups. Let us assume that the survival at study termination in the reference group is 40%, and that the proportion censored (withdrawn) during follow-up is 25% (the `wdprob()` option). If we want a power of 90% to be able to detect a hazard ratio of 0.5 or more extreme, we need 131 participants in each group.

```
. stpower logrank .4, hratio(.5) wdprob(.25) power(.9)
Estimated sample sizes for two-sample comparison of survivor functions
Log-rank test, Freedman method
Ho: S1(t) = S2(t)

Input parameters:

        alpha =     0.0500   (two sided)
           s1 =     0.4000
           s2 =     0.6325
        hratio =     0.5000
        power =     0.9000
           p1 =     0.5000
   withdrawal =       25.00%

Estimated number of events and sample sizes:

            E =          96
            N =         262
           N1 =         131
           N2 =         131
```

`stpower cox` and `stpower exponential` are related commands for more complex scenarios. Again, it may be an advantage to use the dialogs:

```
. db stpower
```

In an FAQ available at http://www.stata.com/support/faqs/stat/power.html, A. Feiveson illustrates how to use simulation techniques to estimate power for a range of regression models (Feiveson 2001). Also see *Stata Journal* papers by Feiveson (2002) and Newson (2004).

16.3   Other analyses

Meta-analysis

Stata has not produced commands specifically aimed at meta-analysis. However, a British group has written several commands aimed at meta-analysis; see Egger, Davey Smith, and Altman (2001). A revised version of the book's chapter about meta-analysis with Stata can (at least as of July 2008) be downloaded from http://www.systematicreviews.com.

Classifying diseases

Facilities for handling diagnostic and procedure codes from ICD-9 (International Classification of Diseases, Ninth Revision) are available with the `icd9` and `icd9p` commands; see [D] **icd9**. Similar facilities for ICD-10 are not available (as of July 2008).

Pharmacokinetic data

The pk family of commands is aimed at analyzing pharmacokinetic data, especially for assessing bioequivalence; see [R] **pk**.

Survey data

The svy family of commands accounts for the sample design in survey studies. Facilities include adjustment for sampling weights, clustering, and stratification. You can find an introduction in [U] **26.17 Survey data** and more detail in the *Survey Data Reference Manual*. See a brief example in section 13.4.

Time-series data

Stata has several commands for analyzing time-series data, which are described in the *Time-Series Reference Manual*.

Panel data

Panel data reflect repeated measurements on individuals or other study objects. Such data have a time structure, and they are clustered in the sense that the measurements on an individual are not independent. The xt family of commands is used for analysis. These commands are described in the *Longitudinal/Panel-Data Reference Manual*. See a brief example in section 13.4.

17 Advanced topics

This chapter discusses several advanced Stata facilities. You may find it useful if you have basic experience and feel a need to go beyond the basics. The chapter is not intended to replace the general manuals. If you are a bit ambitious, you need the *Programming Reference Manual* as well.

17.1 Using saved results

Many Stata commands leave information behind at termination, called *saved results*. Commands such as `predict` and `rvfplot` (section 13.1), `stphplot` and `estat phtest` (section 14.3), `lincom` (section 13.1), and `lroc` (section 15.4) are postestimation commands. They use information (saved results) left by other commands at completion. For an overview, see [U] **20 Estimation and postestimation commands**. For most estimation commands, the *Base Reference Manual* includes a section on postestimation commands, e.g., [R] **logistic postestimation**.

Many users would never wish to know more than this, but if you do, read more about saved results in [U] **18.8 Accessing results calculated by other programs**. If you want to know even more, read [R] **estimates**, [P] **return**, and [P] **ereturn**.

Commands are e-class, r-class, or n-class; n-class commands, such as `generate`, do not save results. We start with the simplest: r-class commands.

Saved results from r-class commands

`summarize` is an r-class command; it saves its results in `r()`. After we run `summarize`, the command `return list` displays the names and contents of the saved results:

```
. cd C:\docs\ishr2
c:\docs\ishr2

. use ras.dta
(Diagnosis of renal artery stenosis)

. summarize crea
```

Variable	Obs	Mean	Std. Dev.	Min	Max
crea	437	93.12815	24.45286	51	189

```
. return list
scalars:
                  r(N) =   437
              r(sum_w) =   437
               r(mean) =   93.12814645308924
                r(Var) =   597.9422564188693
                 r(sd) =   24.45285783745674
                r(min) =   51
                r(max) =   189
                r(sum) =   40697
```

One summarize command can analyze many variables; the saved results refer to the last variable. The saved results can be used by other commands. Here display calculates the standard error from the standard deviation ($r(sd)$) and the number of valid observations ($r(N)$). quietly suppresses the output from summarize, but the results are still saved:

```
. quietly summarize crea
. display "Standard Error = " r(sd)/sqrt(r(N))
Standard Error = 1.1697388
```

The saved results are not part of the dataset but can be considered temporary constants that are available for analysis. They exist until they for some reason disappear, such as when you run another r-class command.

Saved results from e-class commands

Regression analysis commands and several other commands are estimation or e-class commands. These commands save results in e(). Here we use logistic as an example. To see the saved results from an e-class command, use ereturn list:

```
. use ras.dta, clear
(Diagnosis of renal artery stenosis)

. logistic stenosis renogram crea

Logistic regression                             Number of obs   =       437
                                                LR chi2(2)      =    152.91
                                                Prob > chi2     =    0.0000
Log likelihood = -158.59076                     Pseudo R2       =    0.3253
```

stenosis	Odds Ratio	Std. Err.	z	P>|z|	[95% Conf. Interval]	
renogram	17.68998	5.228973	9.72	0.000	9.911079	31.57429
crea	1.017621	.005813	3.06	0.002	1.006291	1.029078

```
. ereturn list
```

scalars:
```
              e(N) =  437
           e(ll_0) =  -235.0458401292179
             e(ll) =  -158.5907608452163
           e(df_m) =  2
           e(chi2) =  152.9101585680031
           e(r2_p) =  .325277312893391
          e(N_cdf) =  0
          e(N_cds) =  0
```

macros:
```
        e(cmdline) : "logistic stenosis renogram crea"
            e(cmd) : "logistic"
        e(predict) : "logistic_p"
          e(title) : "Logistic regression"
            e(vce) : "oim"
         e(depvar) : "stenosis"
       e(crittype) : "log likelihood"
     e(properties) : "b V"
      e(estat_cmd) : "logit_estat"
       e(chi2type) : "LR"
```

matrices:
```
              e(b) :  1 x 3
              e(V) :  3 x 3
          e(rules) :  1 x 4
```

functions:
```
        e(sample)
```

You can find a description of these saved elements in [R] **logistic**.

Postestimation commands such as predict, lincom, and adjust (see sections 13.1, 13.2, and 15.4) use the results saved in e(). If you get the error message last estimates not found, it means that the results needed are not available for some reason, and we must run logistic again. Here we do it quietly to avoid displaying the output again:

```
. lincom renogram + 70*crea + _cons
last estimates not found
r(301);
. quietly logistic stenosis renogram crea
. lincom renogram + 70*crea + _cons
 ( 1)   renogram + 70 crea + _cons = 0
```

stenosis	Odds Ratio	Std. Err.	z	P>|z|	[95% Conf. Interval]	
(1)	1.167837	.3299007	0.55	0.583	.671317	2.031595

lincom itself is an r-class command; it saves in r():

```
. return list
```

scalars:
```
            r(se) =  .3299007364313011
      r(estimate) =  1.167837393719094
```

Information saved in c()

These are not really results, but you can see several Stata settings and constants by typing

```
. creturn list
```

One of the constants displayed is π:

```
...
c(pi) = 3.141592653589793
...
```

The statsby command

statsby (see [D] **statsby**) collects saved results from a command, and it can be done across a by list.

Using the lbw1.dta dataset, we want to create a graph displaying the estimated mean birthweight with confidence intervals for three racial groups. We could obtain the coordinates with

```
. by race, sort: ci bwt
```

and you could enter them with an input command.

statsby uses the results saved after a command, but first we must know their names:

```
. use lbw1.dta
(Hosmer & Lemeshow data)

. ci bwt
    Variable |      Obs       Mean     Std. Err.    [95% Conf. Interval]
-------------+--------------------------------------------------------------
         bwt |      189    2944.286    53.02811      2839.679    3048.892

. return list

scalars:
              r(ub) =  3048.892293354518
              r(lb) =  2839.67913521691
              r(se) =  53.02811244558399
            r(mean) =  2944.285714285714
               r(N) =  189
```

If we are in doubt about the saved results' meaning, we can look up the appropriate manual entry; here it is obvious that we are interested in r(mean), r(ub) (upper 95% confidence limit), and r(lb) (lower 95% confidence limit).

We can now create a new dataset containing three observations (one for each race) and four variables: race, mean birthweight, and lower and upper confidence limits:

```
. statsby mean=r(mean) cil=r(lb) ciu=r(ub), by(race) clear: ci bwt
```
(output omitted)

```
. list
```

	race	mean	cil	ciu
1.	1. white	3103.01	2955.53	3250.491
2.	2. black	2719.692	2461.722	2977.662
3.	3. other	2804.015	2628.076	2979.954

statsby is a prefix command, like by and xi. Here it is a prefix to the ci bwt command that followed the colon. r(mean), etc., are the results saved by ci bwt. The clear option allowed us to overwrite the current dataset.

You can avoid overwriting the current dataset by using the saving() option, as in the following do-file that generates figure 17.1:

─────────────────────────── gph_fig17_1.do ───────────────────────────
```
* gph_fig17_1.do

cd C:\docs\ishr2
use lbw1.dta

statsby mean=r(mean) cil=r(lb) ciu=r(ub), ///
  by(race) saving(bwtrace.dta, replace): ci bwt

use bwtrace.dta, clear
set scheme lean1

twoway                              ///
  (scatter mean race)               ///
  (rcap cil ciu race)               ///
  ,                                 ///
  xtitle("Race")                    ///
  ytitle("Birthweight, grams")      ///
  xscale(range(0.5 3.5))            ///
  xlabel(1 2 3, valuelabel notick)  ///
  legend(off)                       ///
  xsize(3) ysize(2.2) scale(1.4)
```

(Continued on next page)

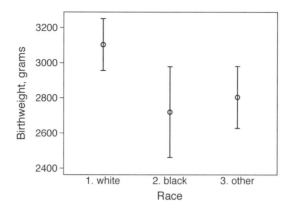

Figure 17.1. `statsby` used to generate coordinates (mean, 95% CI) for a graph

Back in chapter 11, figure 11.32 was created by entering data from a `summarize` output into a do-file with an `input` command. The coordinates can, however, be generated directly from the original data by using `statsby`, as shown in the do-file `gph_fig11_32b.do`, which is not illustrated in this book but available at this book's web site. The data management in this case was quite complex because several variables were involved.

17.2   Macros and scalars

Macros

You can read more about macros in [U] **18.3 Macros** and [P] **macro**.

A Stata macro is a kind of variable that has a name and contents. The content is a character string, but the string may represent a numeric value. A macro is not part of a dataset, but the information is available to the current program or session. In a command including a macro name, the name is replaced by the content before execution. This replacement is called *macro expansion*.

Stata's use of the word *macro* differs from another common usage. *Cambridge Advanced Learner's Dictionary* defines a macro as "a single instruction given to a computer which produces a set of instructions for the computer to perform a particular piece of work". In Stata terminology, this is more like the definition of a program, and Stata macros could have been given the name *micro*.

Local macros live within a program or a session, but only as long as the program or the session is active. Global macros (not to be discussed further here) are those that can be accessed by other programs.

Local macros are typically defined by the `local` command. When used as arguments to other commands, they are put in single quotes, such as `'SE'`. The left single quote is ` (accent grave), and the right quote is the simple ' (apostrophe).

> Here is a hint for producing the left single quote: In this book, the appearance of single quotes differs a bit from how they look on your keyboard and screen. Try `help quotes` to see how they look on your screen. Keyboard layouts differ; on some keyboards, the left single quote is produced by a dead key, meaning that nothing is produced until you press the spacebar.

I chose — although this is not standard — to use capital letters for macro names to distinguish them clearly from variable names.

In section 17.1, we saw the following construct after `summarize` in the `ras.dta` dataset:

```
. quietly summarize crea
. display "Standard Error = " r(sd)/sqrt(r(N))
Standard Error = 1.1697388
```

Now if we want to use the standard error, e.g., for calculating a confidence interval, we must somehow store it. Storing it as a variable in the dataset is not economical because we would have to store as many copies as there are observations. Instead, we store the mean and the standard error as the local macros `MEAN` and `SE`, and we use them to calculate confidence limits:

```
. use ras.dta
(Diagnosis of renal artery stenosis)
. quietly summarize crea
. local SE = r(sd)/sqrt(r(N))
. local MEAN = r(mean)
. display "Mean = " ‘MEAN’ "  SE = " ‘SE’
Mean = 93.128146  SE = 1.1697388
. local CIL = ‘MEAN’ - 1.96*‘SE’
. local CIU = ‘MEAN’ + 1.96*‘SE’
. display "95% CI: " ‘CIL’ " - " ‘CIU’
95% CI: 90.835458 - 95.420835
```

Before execution of the command

```
. local CIL = ‘MEAN’ - 1.96*‘SE’
```

the macro names are replaced by the macro contents. After expansion, the command is

```
. local CIL = 93.128146 - 1.96*1.1697388
```

The macros above contained numerical information. We can also define a local macro directly as a string, without an equal-sign:

```
. local VLIST "stenosis renogram crea"
```

The content of VLIST is the string "stenosis renogram crea". Before execution, the command

```
. logistic ‘VLIST’
```

expands to

```
. logistic stenosis renogram crea
```

This macro could be useful if you are going to perform several analyses using the same list of variables.

A third form of macro comprises extended functions, which use a colon after the macro name. You can read more in [U] **18.3.6 Extended macro functions**. In the following example, the variable label macro function copies the content of the variable label associated with the variable v1 to the macro content:

```
. local LBL : variable label v1
```

At the end of section 17.3, under *Debugging programs*, there is an illustration of macro expansion.

Scalars

Like macros, scalars have a name and contents, and like local macros the information is available to the current program or session. In a macro, the content is a printable string, even if it represents numerical information; scalars contain binary information, and when processing numerical information this is more efficient.

In the example above, we could have used scalars instead of macros. It would have looked like this:

```
. quietly summarize crea
. scalar SE = r(sd)/sqrt(r(N))
. scalar MEAN = r(mean)
. display "Mean = " MEAN "  SE = " SE
Mean = 93.128146  SE = 1.1697388
. scalar CIL = MEAN - 1.96*SE
. scalar CIU = MEAN + 1.96*SE
. display "95% CI: " CIL " - " CIU
95% CI: 90.835458 - 95.420835
```

Unlike macro names, scalar names are not put in quotes, and if a variable and a scalar share a name, Stata will use the information in the variable. As you see, I use uppercase letters for scalar names and lowercase letters for variable names, to avoid mixing them up. Another possibility is to use the scalar() function. You might use it like this:

```
. scalar CIL = scalar(MEAN) - 1.96*scalar(SE)
```

You can read more about scalars in [P] **scalar**.

17.3 Programs

This section shows how you can write your own small programs or commands as ado-files. An ado-file is much like a do-file, but you execute it by calling its name, possibly followed by one or more arguments. The first significant line is a `program` command, and the last is an `end`. The filename must correspond to the name in the `program` command.

To work, an ado-file must be placed in an *ado-path* folder; see section 1.1. Your ado-path folder names are displayed by typing `sysdir`. The folder for your personal creations typically is `C:\ado\personal`, so we will use that in the following discussion.

Imagine that you repeatedly find yourself issuing `list` commands with the options `clean`, `nolabel`, and `noobs` (see section 10.2). Actually, you often forget the options and get frustrated. You can tailor your own command for such listings, calling it, e.g., `mylist`. (First, do a `findit mylist` to make sure that the name does not conflict with existing official or unofficial commands). The simplest possible ado-file would be this `mylist.ado`:

```
                           mylist.ado
program mylist                    // version 1
list, clean noobs nolabel
end
```

Issuing this `mylist` command will make a list of all the variables in all observations, applying the `clean`, `nolabel`, and `noobs` options. You might want more control; `syntax` can help you; see [U] **18.4.4 Parsing standard Stata syntax** and [P] **syntax**. A better version of the program is

```
                           mylist.ado
program mylist                    // version 2
syntax [varlist] [if] [in]
list 'varlist' 'if' 'in', clean noobs nolabel
end
```

Now the command

```
. mylist mpg-weight if price>10000
```

does exactly the same as the command

```
. list mpg-weight if price>10000, clean noobs nolabel
```

This simple example illustrates a strong feature of Stata—you can generate your own commands.

lprob.ado estimates the probability of an outcome

In section 15.4, we used `adjust` after `logistic` to estimate the probability of stenosis, given information on the renography result and the serum-creatinine level. We could have used `adjust` again, but for illustrative purposes, we will instead use `lincom`:

```
. use ras.dta
(Diagnosis of renal artery stenosis)
. quietly logistic stenosis renogram crea
. lincom renogram + 70*crea + _cons
 ( 1)  renogram + 70 crea + _cons = 0
```

stenosis	Odds Ratio	Std. Err.	z	P>|z|	[95% Conf. Interval]	
(1)	1.167837	.3299007	0.55	0.583	.671317	2.031595

Remember that the result of lincom depends on the results saved by the preceding estimation command. Any independent variables included in the logistic command, but not in
the lincom command, are still included — with the value 0. Had we, after the logistic command above, written lincom _cons + renogram, we would get the odds for stenosis among
hypothetical patients with an abnormal renography and a serum-creatinine level of 0.

When including _cons in the arguments for lincom after logistic, the coefficient is an
odds, not an odds ratio as indicated in the heading. To get the corresponding probability, we
type

```
. display 1.167837/2.167837
.53871071
```

If we need to enter this sequence repeatedly, would it not be nice to have a command displaying the probability directly? It certainly would be safer. (Actually, adjust does that for
you, but for now we pretend that it does not.) To illustrate the idea, I created the lprob1 command to be used after logistic. It gives the probability of the outcome with 95% confidence
interval. We do not need to specify _cons; it is included automatically.

```
. lprob1 renogram + 70*crea
 ( 1)  renogram + 70 crea + _cons = 0
```

stenosis	Odds Ratio	Std. Err.	z	P>|z|	[95% Conf. Interval]	
(1)	1.167837	.3299007	0.55	0.583	.671317	2.031595

```
Probability: .53871079     95% CI: .40166702 - .67014287
```

We did this by creating the ado-file C:\ado\personal\lprob1.ado. The first command
in an ado-file is program followed by the program name. The program name must match the
name of the ado-file. The last command is end:

─────────────── C:\ado\personal\lprob1.ado ───────────────
```
program lprob1

lincom '0' + _cons
local LN_0 = ln(r(estimate))
local SE_LN_0 = r(se)/r(estimate)
local CIL = exp('LN_0' - 1.96*'SE_LN_0')
local CIU = exp('LN_0' + 1.96*'SE_LN_0')
local PROB = r(estimate)/(1+r(estimate))
local CIL = 'CIL'/(1 + 'CIL')
local CIU = 'CIU'/(1 + 'CIU')
display " "
display " Probability: " 'PROB' "    95% CI: " 'CIL' " - " 'CIU'

end
```

The information available from `lincom` is the odds for stenosis (`r(estimate)`) and the standard error for odds (`r(se)`). To calculate a confidence interval, we need ln(odds) and SE(ln(odds)). The latter can be calculated by SE(odds)/odds. (The standard error displayed by `lincom` is actually calculated as SE(ln(odds))*odds, so we reverse this calculation.) From ln(odds) and SE(ln(odds)), you can calculate the confidence limits for ln(odds), and from here things are straightforward.

In the second command (`lincom '0' + _cons`) in the above program, the 0 (zero) is a local macro name. It contains whatever was input after the command name; here it was `renogram + 70*crea`. The macro name is put in single quotes, meaning that it will be replaced by its contents before execution. After expansion, the command is

    . lincom renogram + 70*crea + _cons

Next we create the local macro `LN_0`. It contains the result of the expression `ln(r(estimate))`, i.e., ln(odds).

`r(se)` is another saved result from `lincom`; it is the standard error of the estimate. We calculate SE(ln(odds)) and assign the result to the local macro `SE_LN_0`.

The content of local macro `CIL` is the lower 95% confidence limit for the odds — same procedure for the upper limit.

Let local macro `PROB` contain the probability: odds/(1+odds). Replace the values in `CIL` and `CIU` in the same way.

The following version of `lprob.ado` includes comments and aims to be fail-safe.

(Continued on next page)

```
───────────────────── C:\ado\personal\lprob.ado ─────────────────────
*! lprob ver 1.0 27apr2005
*! Calculates probability of outcome after -logistic- or -logit-.
*! Author: Svend Juul
  program lprob
  version 9

* Check that we have saved results from -logistic- or -logit-
  if "`e(cmd)'" != "logistic" & "`e(cmd)'" != "logit" {
     display as error "lprob only works after -logistic- or -logit-"
     error 301
  }

* If no arguments, include _cons.
* If _cons is specified, don't include it again;
* otherwise include it.
  if "`0'" == "" {                                     // No arguments
     quietly lincom _cons, or
  }
  else if strpos("`0'","_cons") {                      // _cons specified
     quietly lincom `0', or
  }
  else {                                               // None of the above
     quietly lincom `0' + _cons, or
  }

  local LN_O = ln(r(estimate))                         // ln(odds)
  local SE_LN_O = r(se)/r(estimate)                    // SE(ln(odds))

* Instead of 1.96, use the more precise invnormal(0.975)
  local CIL = exp(`LN_O' - invnormal(0.975)*`SE_LN_O') // CI for odds
  local CIU = exp(`LN_O' + invnormal(0.975)*`SE_LN_O') // CI for odds
  local PROB = r(estimate)/(1 + r(estimate))           // Probability
  local CIL = `CIL'/(1 + `CIL')                        // CI for probability
  local CIU = `CIU'/(1 + `CIU')                        // CI for probability

* We want the dependent variable's label in output.
  local VARLAB : variable label `e(depvar)'

* If the dependent variable has no label, don't try to include it;
* if it has, include it in parenthesis.
  display " "

  if "`VARLAB'" == "" {                                // No variable label
     display as result "Probability of `e(depvar)':"
  }
  else {                                               // Variable label
     display as result "Probability of `e(depvar)' (`VARLAB'):"
  }
```

```
display as result ///
    %08.6f 'PROB' " (95% CI: " %08.6f 'CIL' " - " %08.6f 'CIU' ")"

end
```

This is the final version of the lprob program, and the output looks like this:

```
. lprob renogram + 70*crea
Probability of stenosis (Stenosis at angiography):
0.538711 (95% CI: 0.401669 - 0.670141)
```

If an ado-file is of more permanent value—especially if it might be used by others—it should have a header with a short description. If you want quick information about a command, use the which command:

```
. which lprob
C:\ado\plus\l\lprob.ado
*! lprob ver 1.0 27apr2005
*! Calculates probability of outcome after -logistic- or -logit-.
*! Author: Svend Juul
```

This program has been tested with Stata version 9; if you try to run it with version 8, it might malfunction. version 9 will, therefore, give an error message if you try it with version 8. In future Stata versions, some functionalities might change, but typing version 9 ensures that the program will still be working. The rest of the program is probably self-explanatory.

Having created a program that might be useful to others, you may want to make it public at the SSC archives; see section 2.2. You also must create a help-file; see [U] **18.11.6 Writing online help**.

After I developed the lprob program, I discovered that the adjust command does what I wanted. I decided, however, to keep the description of lprob to illustrate the development of an ado-file. Like lincom, adjust is a postestimation command. Running it after a logistic command with the pr and ci options, we get the following:

```
. quietly logistic stenosis renogram crea
. adjust renogram=1 crea=70, pr ci
```

```
      Dependent variable: stenosis     Command: logistic
      Covariates set to value: renogram = 1, crea = 70
```

All	pr	lb	ub
	.538711	[.401669	.670141]

```
Key:  pr        =  Probability
      [lb , ub] =  [95% Confidence Interval]
```

Debugging programs

If a program is interrupted by an error message, we cannot see which program line created the error. We might also have a program that does not give the result intended. For example, a previous version of lprob was lprob2:

```
───────────────────── C:\ado\personal\lprob2.ado ─────────────────
program lprob2

lincom '0' + _cons
local LN_0 = ln(r(estimate))
local SE_LN_0 = r(se)/r(estimate)
local CIL = exp('LN_0' - 1.96*'SE_LN_0')
local CIU = exp('LN_0' + 1.96*'SE_LN_0')
local PROB = r(estimate)/(1+r(estimate))
local CIL = 'CIL'/(1 + 'CIL')
local CIU = 'CIU'/(1 + 'CIU')
display " "
display " Probability: " 'PROB' "     95% CI: " 'CIL' " - " 'CIU'

end
```

Running it gives the following output:

```
. lprob2 renogram + 70*crea

 ( 1)  renogram + 70 crea + _cons = 0
```

stenosis	Odds Ratio	Std. Err.	z	P>|z|	[95% Conf. Interval]	
(1)	1.167837	.3299007	0.55	0.583	.671317	2.031595

```
96* invalid name
r(198);
```

I had difficulty locating the error. However, with

```
. set trace on
```

all program lines will be displayed, including other programs called by the program. The amount of output may be overwhelming, but you can restrict it by typing

```
. set tracedepth 1
```

Comparing the expanded commands with your expectations can give you a clue:

```
. set trace on
. set tracedepth 1
. lprob2 renogram + 70*crea
```

```
                                                    ─── begin lprob2 ───
- lincom '0' + _cons
= lincom renogram + 70*crea + _cons

 ( 1)  renogram + 70 crea + _cons = 0
```

stenosis	Odds Ratio	Std. Err.	z	P>|z|	[95% Conf. Interval]	
(1)	1.167837	.3299007	0.55	0.583	.671317	2.031595

```
- local LN_O = ln(r(estimate))
- local SE_LN_O = r(se)/r(estimate)
- local CIL = exp('LN_O' - 1.96*'SE_LN_0')
= local CIL = exp(.1551536570080954 - 1.96*)
96* invalid name
                                                    ─── end lprob2 ───
r(198);
```

For lines including a macro, you first see the original program line, preceded by $-$, and next the expanded command, preceded by $=$:

```
- lincom '0' + _cons
= lincom renogram + 70*crea + _cons
```

Looking at

```
- local CIL = exp('LN_O' - 1.96*'SE_LN_0')
= local CIL = exp(.1551536570080954 - 1.96*)
96* invalid name
```

you discover that 'SE_LN_0' expanded to nothing. This is a common mistake: the macro name should be SE_LN_O (capital O), but I had written SE_LN_0 (zero). Now let's correct the error. Remember we need to set trace off before proceeding. Read more about debugging in [P] **trace**.

17.4 Useful programming commands

The term *programming commands* does not mean that the commands can be used only in programs, i.e., ado-files. They can also be used in do-files and even interactively. The following commands are documented in the *Programming Reference Manual* ([P]).

if ... else if ... else

Do not confuse the if *command* with the if *qualifier* (section 4.4). The if qualifier asks questions about the data for each observation (... if crea < 70), and this leads to selection of the observations to be processed. The if command asks questions about the command environment, e.g., the contents of a certain macro, and this leads to selecting commands to be used on all observations, as in

```
if "'0'" == "" {                        // No arguments specified
   quietly lincom _cons, or
}
else if strpos("'0'","_cons") {        // _cons specified
   quietly lincom '0', or
}
else {                                  // None of the above
   quietly lincom '0' + _cons, or
}
```

The meaning of the else if and else commands should be obvious. The braces must be used exactly as shown: the opening brace, {, comes at the end of the command, and the closing brace, }, on a line of its own. The purpose of the indentation is to improve legibility; it means nothing to Stata. When there is only one command between the braces, you can omit them, and you thus could have written the above construct as

```
if "'0'" == "" quietly lincom _cons, or
else if strpos("'0'","_cons") quietly lincom '0', or
else quietly lincom '0' + _cons, or
```

foreach

Section 10.3 demonstrates a shortcoming of tab2. If we want a cross-tabulation of one variable with several other variables, we must give as many commands as we want tables. Here we want a cross-tabulation of each of the variables q1-q10 with treat. The foreach command solves the problem:

```
foreach Q of varlist q1-q10 {
   tab2 'Q' treat
}
```

The local macro Q is a stand-in for q1 to q10, and the construct generates 10 commands:

```
tab2 q1 treat

tab2 q2 treat

...
```

foreach commands can be nested, and you could create a cross-tabulation for each of the variables r1-r5 with each of the variables c1-c10 (a total of 50 tables):

```
foreach R of varlist r1-r5 {
   foreach C of varlist c1-c10 {
      tab2 'R' 'C'
   }
}
```

Although foreach is described in the *Programming Reference Manual*, it can be used as an ordinary command in do-files as well, and even interactively by typing the commands directly into the Command window. In the following do-file, we create 5 observations with 5 variables containing random numbers between 0 and 1:

```
clear
set obs 5
foreach Q of newlist q1-q5 {
    generate 'Q' = uniform()
}
list
```

When you run the do-file, the output looks like this with the commands numbered within the foreach loop:

```
. clear

. set obs 5
obs was 0, now 5

. foreach Q of newlist q1-q5 {
  2.     generate 'Q' = uniform()
  3. }

. list
```

	q1	q2	q3	q4	q5
1.	.0264971	.8116255	.0522238	.1895829	.9307174
2.	.1727387	.1745866	.349758	.0624414	.3240527
3.	.0292306	.2453097	.5232757	.1508073	.4708069
4.	.7537692	.1119462	.3259046	.577387	.3824427
5.	.6555921	.7595286	.2854945	.958726	.6267027

The rules for the placement of braces are the same as for if. foreach takes different types of lists; read more in [P] **foreach** or help foreach. Above you saw varlist referring to existing variables and newlist referring to variables to be created. numlist refers to a numeric list; see the example in the next section (forvalues).

forvalues

forvalues lets you loop over a numeric range. The following trivial example illustrates the principle:

```
. forvalues I = 1/3 {
  2.     display 'I'
  3. }
1
2
3
```

The numeric range can be specified as shown, or as, e.g., (0(5)25), but not all numeric list forms (see section 4.3) are allowed; see [P] **forvalues** or help forvalues. If you want to loop over the values 4, 3, 2, 7, 6, 5, 4, 3, 2, 1, then a standard numeric list could be 4/2 7/1, but forvalues will give an error message:

```
. forvalues I = 4/2 7/1 {
  2.    display 'I'
  3. }
invalid syntax
r(198);
```

You can solve this problem by using `foreach` with `numlist`, which accepts standard numeric lists, such as

```
. foreach I of numlist 4/2 7/1 {
  2.    display 'I'
  3. }
4
3
2
7
```
  (output omitted)

Parallel lists

If you have experience with Stata version 7 and earlier, you might recall the `for` command, which has been removed in favor of `foreach` and `forvalues`. One of the nice things about it, however, was its ability to handle parallel lists. Below I show how this can be obtained by using `forvalues`; see a cute FAQ (http://www.stata.com/support/faqs/lang/parallel.html) and a paper by Cox (2003a) for more information.

Let's say we have the variables x1-x5 and y1-y5, and we want to generate the variables z1-z5, where z1=x1*y1, z2=x2*y2, etc. The values of the primary variables are

```
. list
```

	x1	x2	x3	x4	x5	y1	y2	y3	y4	y5
1.	0	8	1	2	9	9	10	7	7	4
2.	2	2	3	1	3	1	0	0	5	5
3.	0	2	5	2	5	1	4	10	1	6
4.	8	1	3	6	4	5	3	7	9	0
5.	7	8	3	10	6	1	6	3	1	0

With `forvalues`, we can do the following:

```
. forvalues I=1/5 {            // I takes the values 1,2,3,4,5
  2.    generate z'I' = x'I' * y'I'   // z-variables are the products:
  3. }                         // z1=x1*y1, z2=x2*y2, etc.
. list
```

	x1	x2	x3	x4	x5	y1	y2	y3	y4	y5	z1	z2	z3	z4	z5
1.	0	8	1	2	9	9	10	7	7	4	0	80	7	14	36
2.	2	2	3	1	3	1	0	0	5	5	2	0	0	5	15
3.	0	2	5	2	5	1	4	10	1	6	0	8	50	2	30
4.	8	1	3	6	4	5	3	7	9	0	40	3	21	54	0
5.	7	8	3	10	6	1	6	3	1	0	7	48	9	10	0

The structure of variable names made the solution rather simple, but what if the variables are a-e and p-t, and we want to generate the variables ap=a*p, bq=b*q, etc.? The primary variables are

```
. list
```

	a	b	c	d	e	p	q	r	s	t
1.	0	8	1	2	9	9	10	7	7	4
2.	2	2	3	1	3	1	0	0	5	5
3.	0	2	5	2	5	1	4	10	1	6
4.	8	1	3	6	4	5	3	7	9	0
5.	7	8	3	10	6	1	6	3	1	0

The trick is to use describe with the varlist option (see [D] **describe**). It saves a list of variable names in r(varlist), and the lists are assigned to the local macros XVARS and YVARS:

```
. quietly describe a-e, varlist    // list variable names a-e to r(varlist)
. local XVARS "'r(varlist)'"        // local macro XVARS contains variable names
. quietly describe p-t, varlist    // list variable names p-t to r(varlist)
. local YVARS "'r(varlist)'"        // local macro YVARS contains variable names
```

Next take the pairs of variables to be multiplied, using the extended macro function word ... of to pick variables sequentially (see [U] **18.3.6 Extended macro functions**):

```
. forvalues I=1/5 {                   // I takes the values 1,2,3,4,5
  2.    local X : word 'I' of 'XVARS' // Assign the Ith word of "a b c d e"
                                       //    to macro X
  3.    local Y : word 'I' of 'YVARS' // Assign the Ith word of "p q r s t"
                                       //    to macro Y
  4.    generate 'X''Y' = 'X' * 'Y'   // variable XY is the product of two
                                       //    variables:
  5. }                                 // ap=a*p, bq=b*q, etc.
. list
```

	a	b	c	d	e	p	q	r	s	t	ap	bq	cr	ds	et
1.	0	8	1	2	9	9	10	7	7	4	0	80	7	14	36
2.	2	2	3	1	3	1	0	0	5	5	2	0	0	5	15
3.	0	2	5	2	5	1	4	10	1	6	0	8	50	2	30
4.	8	1	3	6	4	5	3	7	9	0	40	3	21	54	0
5.	7	8	3	10	6	1	6	3	1	0	7	48	9	10	0

(Continued on next page)

Other commands

`continue` within a `foreach` or `forvalues` loop returns control to the `foreach` or `forvalues` command, thus skipping the remaining commands in the current loop iteration. `continue, break` jumps to the next command after the loop. See [P] **continue** for more information on `continue`.

```
forvalues I = 1/1000 {
    if 'I' > 100 {
        continue, break
    }
    display 'I' "  " sqrt('I')
}
```

`capture` can be used in do-files and ado-files to allow the job to continue despite an erroneous command; the standard behavior is that the job is terminated. It can be used, for example, to generate specific error messages (although this one is not that specific). `_rc` is an error code that reflects the error status of the last command; it is 0 if the command is valid. See [P] **capture** for more information about `capture`.

```
capture summarize var1
if _rc != 0 {
    display as error "Variable does not exist"
}
```

17.5   Do-files and ado-files useful for handling output

Elaborate profile.do

In chapter 1, you saw a simple `profile.do`, which automatically opens an output log file (`stata.log`) and a command log file (`cmdlog.txt`) at the start of a session. Here is a more elaborate version that adds a time stamp to the command log file, which will make it easier for you to reconstruct previous work. `profile.do` puts the log files in `C:\` (the root folder), but of course you may decide to put them elsewhere.

The time stamp is created using the c-class date and time macros. You may include a DOS command by prefixing it with `shell` or `!`; see [D] **shell**.

```
━━━━━━━━━━━━━━━━━━ C:\ado\personal\profile.do ━━━━━━━━━━━━━━━━━━
* C:\ado\personal\profile.do  executes automatically when opening Stata.

* Write session start time in time.txt.
  set obs 2
  gen time="******* Session started: `c(current_date)'  `c(current_time)'"
  replace time=" " if _n==1
  outfile time using "C:\time.txt", noquote replace
  clear

* Copy session start time to the cmdlog (cmdlog.txt) and open it.
* ! means that a DOS command follows.
  ! copy  /b  C:\cmdlog.txt + C:\time.txt  C:\cmdlog.txt  /y
  cmdlog using "C:\cmdlog.txt", append

* Open the output log in text format (stata.log)
* for display in a text editor or the Viewer.
  log using "C:\stata.log", replace

* If you want an output log in smcl format (stata.smcl)
* for display in the Viewer, replace the above line with:
*    log using "C:\stata.smcl", replace
```

Ado-files for handling output

If you have an active output log, *Ctrl+L* lets you view it in the Viewer, or suspend or close it. This method will work regardless of the name and type (text or SMCL) of your output log.

Your output log may have become large, so suppose you want to start a fresh log. The `newlog` command lets you do that. The content of a minimal `newlog.ado` is

```
━━━━━━━━━━━━━━━━━━━━━━ newlog.ado ━━━━━━━━━━━━━━━━━━━━━━
program newlog
log close
log using C:\stata.log, replace
end
```

The above ado-file will work, but it can be improved:

(Continued on next page)

```
                          ──────── newlog.ado ────────
*! newlog ver 1.0 30jul2005
*! Closes current output log and opens a new output log.
*! Author: Svend Juul

program define newlog
version 9
args LOG
if "`LOG'" != "" {
  capture log close
  log using "`LOG'", replace
}
else {
  quietly log
  local LOG "`r(filename)'"
  if "`LOG'" == "" {
    log using C:\stata.log, replace
  }
  else {
    log close
    log using "`LOG'", replace
  }
}

end
```

newlog may be called with a log filename, in which case the current log, if any, is closed and a new log with the specified filename opens:

. **newlog mylog.log**

If you call newlog without a filename, it examines whether a log is open, in which case it is replaced by a new log with the same name. Otherwise, the text output log C:\stata.log is opened.

You can use the Viewer (*Ctrl+L*) to inspect a snapshot of the output log, and you can use the mouse to select part of it for printing or for copying to another document. The Viewer can display both plain text logs and SMCL-formatted logs.

As a general rule, log files from important analyses or data management tasks should not be tampered with, but sometimes you need to keep the valid parts and discard the invalid parts of the output; you may also need to add explanatory comments to the results. For such tasks, I prefer using a general text editor to inspect and modify output before printing. Compared to using the Viewer window, you have more freedom, and you can edit it by using the mouse or the keyboard. This method requires a text output log. My favorite text editor, NoteTab Light, can be downloaded for free. You can find a short description and a link to its web site at my web site; see *Other supplementary materials provided by the author* at http://www.stata-press.com/books/ishr2.html.

nlog opens a copy of the output log in NoteTab Light. The content of nlog.ado is

```
——————————————————————— nlog.ado ———————————————————

*! nlog ver 1.0 27apr2005
*! Opens output log in NoteTab Light
*! Author: Svend Juul

program nlog
version 9
quietly log

if "'r(filename)'" == "" {
   display as error "No log file"
}
else {
   winexec "C:\Program files\NoteTab Light\NoteTab.exe" "'r(filename)'"
}

end
```

The Stata command winexec executes a Windows command. Obviously, you need to check where NoteTab Light was installed and modify nlog.ado accordingly.

The above profile.do and ado-files are available at this book's web site, http://www.stata-press.com/books/ishr2.html. profile.do is downloaded to the same folder as the datasets and other do-files; from here you should copy it to C:\ado\personal if you want to make it work. You should read through profile.do to see if you want to use it as is or if you need to modify it for your particular Stata and computer configuration.

The ado-files are typically downloaded to C:\ado\plus.

18 Taking good care of your data

The purpose of this chapter is to give some preventive advice: how to protect yourself against mistakes, errors, loss of data, and wasted time. Avoiding these pitfalls requires you to work systematically and pay consistent attention to documentation issues. A more elaborate version of this chapter can be found in the web book *Take Good Care of Your Data* (Juul 2005); see *Other supplementary materials provided by the author* at http://www.stata-press.com/books/ishr2.html.

I have seen quite a few accidents with data—including some where I had only myself to blame—that could have been prevented with modest investments in documentation and safeguards. These were accidents such as

- Not being able to reconstruct a published result.

- Not being able to explain why the number of participants in the dataset was 157; it ought to have been 159.

- Having trouble understanding your own data when you return to them after a 4-week break.

- Making a mistake on how data were coded, thus arriving at an erroneous result.

- Working on the wrong dataset.

- Not being able to restore archived data (they were on a tape that no existing tape drive could read).

- Having taken careful backup—and storing the backup media in the same room as the computer (the office burned).

Such incidents at least lead to wasted time and sometimes the consequences are much worse. But prevention is not that difficult.

18.1 The audit trail

When keeping financial accounts, such as for a company or an association, there are some obvious principles to follow.

It must be possible to go back from the balance sheet to the individual vouchers. This is done by giving each voucher a unique number. From each item in the balance sheet, you must be able to identify the component amounts and the corresponding vouchers. The term *audit trail* means that, from the final results, you must be able to follow the trail backward to the primary sources of information. If you are the bookkeeper, you need this for yourself; otherwise, you will have a hard time tracing errors. And it is mandatory for auditing.

The same principles apply when handling information in research. You should be able to trace each piece of information back to the original source document:

- ID (case identifier) must be included in the original documents and in the dataset.
- All corrections must be documented and explained.
- All modifications to the dataset must be documented by do-files.
- All major analyses must be documented by do-files.

This technique is needed during error checking and correction, when generating new variables, and when your project is exposed to external audit and monitoring.

The purposes are primarily to protect yourself against mistakes, errors, wasted time, and loss of information, and secondarily to enable external audit. Documentation procedures must be included during project planning, and they should be with you all the time.

18.2   Data collection

The design of your data collection instruments like questionnaires and case report forms can have strong implications for the quality of your data. For some advice, see Juul (2005). You might search the Internet by using keywords such as "questionnaire layout" to find more advice. I found one that I like from the University of Leeds at
http://www.leeds.ac.uk/iss/documentation/top/top2.pdf.

With questionnaires, there are two important considerations:

- The respondent: the questionnaire should be designed to minimize the risk of mistakes and errors.
- The data processing: the questionnaire should be easy to handle, and the risk of coding and transcription errors should be minimized.

The first consideration is by far the most important, as there is no way to correct a respondent's mistakes afterward.

Collect and record raw, not processed, information

Avoid grouping continuous information at data collection time. For example, it is just as easy for the respondent to state her age in years as it is to choose between age groups. Even better, the date of birth allows the computer to calculate the exact age at any other time.

18.3   The codebook

The codebook is the link between the original data and the data entered in the computer, and it should be prepared early in the process. Here is a short example:

Variable	Source	Meaning	Codes, valid range	Format[a]
id	Q1	Questionnaire number	1–750	3.0
sex	Q2	Respondent's sex	1 Male 2 Female 9 No response	1.0
byear	Q3	Year of birth	1890–1990 -2^b No response	4.0
schooled	Q4	Left school, level	1 Before finishing 9th 2 After 9th 3 After 10th 4 After high school 5 Other 9 No response	1.0
children	Q5	No. of children	0–10 -2^b No response	2.0
voced	Q6	Vocational education	1 None 2 Manual, <3 years 3 Manual, 3 years + 4 Nonmanual, <3 years 5 Nonmanual, 3–4 years 6 Nonmanual, 5 years + 7 Cannot be classified 9 No response	1.0
init	Q7	Initials	Max. 3 initials	A3

[a] This notation is often used when describing formats. 2.0 means a numerical variable with two digits and no decimals. 5.2 means five digits, including a decimal period and two decimals. A3 means a 3-character string (text) variable. You might use Stata's format descriptors instead, such as %3.0f and %3s.

[b] Missing values for interval-scale variables should not be included in calculations.

Codes

Standard recommendation is to always use numerical codes. Not all analyses can handle string codes (e.g., "M" for male sex), and numerical codes are faster to enter and easier to handle during analysis. For interval-scale variables (year of birth, number of children), just use the value as the code, and state the possible range in the codebook. For categorical variables (sex, education), state the meaning of each code. This information should be included in the dataset as value labels.

For open questions, the text information should not be entered as it is in the computer, but you must translate the text into a finite number of categories. The categories should be described in the codebook. Add a coding field next to the response field, and design it so that it does not confuse respondents. Before deciding on a final classification, you might want to classify a sample of, for example, 100 responses to see if it works.

People do not always fill in questionnaires as you expect. Say you asked about cups of coffee per day and expected a single number, but you got responses like "2–3" and "2–4". For such situations, devise a rule, such as "Calculate the average and round up if necessary". The codes for missing values require special attention; see section 5.3.

18.4   Folders and filenames: The log book

Sections 18.5–18.7 illustrate the steps from data entry to a final dataset for analysis. In your own research, there may be more steps, so there is good reason to plan ahead. Here is some advice on decisions that should be made early.

Choose which folder to use for the project

My advice is to organize your folders by subject, not by file type. For a specific project or subproject, keep all your main text files, data files, and do-files in the same folder; an illustration is shown in chapter 21. Do not mix files from different projects in the same folder. Take a copy of the final data and do-files, and put them in a "safe" folder.

Never put your own files in a program folder. You may never find them again, or they may be destroyed if you upgrade the program.

Decide on a system for naming your data and do-files

Do-files that add modifications to your data are vital documentation. It is tempting to issue single commands, one at a time, but it is a lot safer to create a do-file with all the commands needed and execute them together—in the right sequence. You will make errors while developing a do-file, but in the end you will succeed, and you should, of course, keep only the correct do-files for documentation. The vital do-files should include everything needed—but nothing else—to reconstruct the data from the original input.

These do-files should have names clearly indicating what they do. I offer the suggestion to let such do-files start with gen_, followed by the name of the result file. Do-files that do not create new versions of the data should not have this prefix. You can use a different system, but without a system you risk confusion. The log book illustrates my suggestion for naming the data and do-files used in sections 18.6–18.7.

Choose a system for variable names

If you have only a few variables, use names that give intuitive meaning, as in section 18.3 about codebooks. If you have a lot of variables, instead use names derived from, e.g., question numbers: q7a, q7b, etc.; an intuitive system will break down for you. In complex projects where you have data from several sources, use variable names that reflect the source. If you have three interviews with the same people, use the prefixes a, b, c:

```
1st interview:    a1 a2 a3a a3b a3c ...
2nd interview:    b1 b2 ...
```

Keep a log book—and keep it updated

To review your past actions, keep a log book and update it whenever you add modifications to your data. This log book corresponds to the data modifications performed in sections 18.6–18.7.

Project: Treatment of diseaseX
Working folder: `C:\docs\disx`
Safe folder: `C:\docs\disx\safe`

Input data	Do-file	Output data	Comments

visit1a2.rec
visit1a.rec
 	
(EpiData files)
	exported from
	EpiData
		visit1a.dta	12 oct 2004
			Final comparison of two
			   corrected data entry files.
			Agreement documented in
			   `visit1_compare.txt`

visit1a.dta	gen_visit1b.do	visit1b.dta	13 oct 2004 Add labels to `visit1a.dta`
visit1b.dta	gen_visit1c.do	visit1c.dta	15 oct 2004 Identified errors corrected (see `visit1_correct.doc`)
visit1c.dta visit2c.dta	gen_visit12.do	visit12.dta	16 oct 2004 Merging data from visit 1 and visit 2
visit12.dta	gen_visit12a.do	visit12a.dta	16 oct 2004 Generate new variables: `hrqol, opagr`

Make a master do-file

I recommend making a master do-file corresponding to the log book. This file is just a series of do commands that ensures that you perform tasks in the right sequence. Imagine that you discovered an error when analyzing data. You could now incorporate the correction in gen_visit1c.do, and from the master do-file, run it and the subsequent do-files again:

```
―――――――――――――――― master.do ――――――――――――――――
* master.do
cd C:\docs\disx
* Add labels
do gen_visit1b.do
* Correct errors
do gen_visit1c.do
* Merge data from visit 1 and visit 2
do gen_visit12.do
* Generate new variables
do gen_visit12a.do
```

Instead of using the cd command, we could have defined the full path for each file. The important thing is to define the path, one way or the other:

```
―――――――――――――――― master.do ――――――――――――――――
* master.do
* Add labels
do C:\docs\disx\gen_visit1b.do
* Correct errors
do C:\docs\disx\gen_visit1c.do
* Merge data from visit 1 and visit 2
do C:\docs\disx\gen_visit12.do
* Generate new variables
do C:\docs\disx\gen_visit12a.do
```

18.5 Entering data

With small datasets, we can enter data in Stata's Data Editor, but with larger datasets this method is cumbersome and prone to error. Instead, use a data entry program such as EpiData; see section 6.2. You can also find a short description of EpiData and a link to its web site from the author's web site; see *Other supplementary materials provided by the author* at http://www.stata-press.com/books/ishr2.html. EpiData can be downloaded for free.

Preparations

Before entering data, you need to have a complete codebook. All decisions on coding should be made — and documented in the codebook — before you enter data; otherwise, the risk of errors increases.

Examine the source documents (e.g., questionnaires) for obvious inconsistencies before you enter data. Do any coding of text information before, not during, data entry, and write it in the source document.

When defining the dataset, you need the codebook information on variable names and formats (the number of digits needed to represent the information).

Especially when you have data from several sources, you need to write down a plan for the process, including the folder structure, filenames, and variable names. Also make a plan on how to back up your work to reduce the consequences of human, software, or hardware errors; see section 18.9.

Error prevention

A good data entry program such as EpiData enables you to create forms resembling your questionnaire or case-report form pages. This reduces the risk of misplacing information during data entry. "Parallel shifting" during data entry is a common source of error. Parallel shifting is when a correct value is entered, but in the wrong place.

If you enter the wrong ID number, it may be hard to locate and correct the error. I suggest that you reenter the ID number as the last field in the data entry form as a safeguard.

EpiData lets you specify valid values and value labels for each variable. You then get a warning during data entry if you enter an outlier. While this method identifies illegal values, it does not catch erroneous entries within the legal range. You may also specify extended checks, for example, if a date of hospital admission is after the date of birth. However, specifying the rules correctly may be time-consuming, and incorrect specifications will interfere with data entry. Also, inconsistent responses—which can be quite frequent—can interfere with data entry. I prefer to check for illegal values later; see section 18.6.

EpiData lets you enter data twice (preferably by two different operators) and compare the contents of the two files to get a list of discrepancies. Examine the original source documents, and decide which entry was correct. Correct the errors in both files, and run a new comparison, which should show no errors. Keep this output as documentation that the dataset is "clean".

Proofreading is a rather inefficient (and boring) way of error checking and is virtually impossible for large data volumes. At the very least, you need an assistant and a printout of the data entered. Proofreading data on the screen is especially inefficient and will strain your eyes.

Which level of safeguards should you use?

Use cost–benefit thinking. If you made a clinical trial with $50 + 50$ patients, the extra cost of double data entry is much lower than the total cost of collecting the information, and one error might affect the conclusion. You should do everything to avoid errors in your data. If, on the other hand, you mailed a questionnaire to 10,000 people to estimate the prevalence of certain conditions, the consequence of one error is small, and you might decide to save the cost of double entry of every questionnaire.

Modern ways of entering data

Using optical reading is smart for large numbers of small questionnaires (such as the pools). For small numbers of large questionnaires, using optical reading is highly inefficient because of the time spent with preparations. The first consideration is to the respondent, but the layout requirements for optical reading may counteract this consideration.

Especially with telephone interviews, it might be practical to enter responses directly into the computer during the interview, thus avoiding the paper step. This is a good idea for simple mass surveys and opinion polls. For other research purposes, it may not be worth the investment because setting up a correct form for data entry might be quite time-consuming, and if an unpredicted situation arises during an interview, you might get stuck. You will need a lot of experience to be able to do that.

18.6   Inspecting and correcting your data

With complex datasets, you should examine and make corrections to each partial dataset before merging files. In the following examples, there are two partial datasets: `visit1` and `visit2`.

Adding labels to your data

You should define variables and value labels (see section 7.1) in the codebook before you enter data, and EpiData can include them in the dataset before the data is entered. You might, however, have received the raw data from another source. In that case, you should define labels now, before examining the results. Stata does not need the labels, but you need them for readable output.

`gen_visit1b.do` is the do-file that generates the `visit1b.dta` dataset:

```
———————————————————— gen_visit1b.do ————————————————————
* gen_visit1b.do generates visit1b.dta - 12 oct 2004
* Adding labels to primary data

cd C:\docs\disx
use visit1a.dta

label variable id "Questionnaire number"
label variable sex "Sex of respondent"
label variable byear "Year of birth"
...
label define sexlbl  1 "male"  2 "female"
label values sex sexlbl
...
recode byear (9999=.a)
numlabel, add

save visit1b.dta
```

This do-file includes vital documentation and should be saved and kept in a safe place. It starts with reading the input data file and ends with saving the modified dataset. I strongly recommend giving the do-file a name that tells what it does. For example, gen_visit1b.do generates the visit1b.dta dataset. Include the do-file's name as a comment in the first line.

The value 9999 was entered for missing year of birth. This code was recoded to Stata's user-defined missing code, .a. Stata does not display the codes and the value labels simultaneously in output, but the numlabel command incorporates the numeric codes in the value labels.

Searching for errors

After adding labels to your data, print a compact codebook as an overview of your variables, and simple frequency tables of appropriate variables:

```
. use visit1b.dta
. describe
. codebook, compact
. label list occup
. tab1 sex nation-educ
. tab2 sex pregnant
```

describe and codebook give an overview of your variables. Look for the minimum, maximum, and number of valid values in the codebook output. label list shows value-label lists.

tab1 shows tables for all variables mentioned (avoid tables for variables with many values). tab2 can disclose inconsistent information (such as pregnant males).

Because this job did not modify your data, you need not save the commands as a do-file for documentation. You can save it, but do not give it the gen prefix because it does not generate new data.

You should make a printout of the tables produced; do not use the screen. You can easily miss an error — and strain your eyes. Examine the following:

- Compare the codebook created with your original codebook (section 18.3), and check that you made the label information correctly.
- Inspect the overview table (codebook, compact), especially for illegal or improbable minimum and maximum values. Also check that the number of valid observations for each variable is as expected.
- Inspect the frequency tables (tab1) for strange values and for values that should have labels but do not.
- Examine tables that could indicate inconsistencies (such as pregnant males).

If you identified any suspicious values, list them with the ID number (which must also be written at the source document's front page) and check them.

Data entry errors sometimes occur if you misplace the values entered. If you discover an error, also proofread the neighboring variables because they will have a high risk of errors, too. In the following commands, byear-diag represents sex and its neighbors; age1-educ represents pregnant and its neighbors:

```
. use visit1b.dta
. list id byear-diag if sex>2, nolabel
. list id byear-diag age1-educ if sex==1 & pregnant==1, nolabel
```

Make a printout of the lists created; do not use the screen. Next go back to the original documents, identify the errors, and write the corrections on the lists. Examine the neighboring variables carefully because they have a high risk of error, too.

Correction of errors

If you discover an error, you might intuitively go to the Data Editor and correct it there, but I discourage this method. First, the risk of "correcting" the wrong variable or observation is high. Second, the change will be poorly documented, breaking the audit trail.

You should make corrections in a do-file. The gen prefix indicates that this do-file generates a new version of the dataset.

```
                        ─── gen_visit1c.do ───
* gen_visit1c.do
* Corrections 14 oct 2004. See project log page 27.

cd C:\docs\disx
use visit1b.dta
replace sex=2 if id==2473
replace weight=75 if id==3771
...

save visit1c.dta
```

In this way, you have full documentation of the changes made to the dataset, and the audit trail is not broken.

On the other hand, if you discover errors when comparing files after double data entry, you can make corrections directly in the data entered, provided that you end this step with a new comparison of the corrected files and, it is hoped, demonstrate that there are no disagreements. The point is that you split the process in distinct and well-defined steps and that your documentation from one step to the next is consistent. But you should not bother documenting that you made and corrected errors during the data entry, any more than I should document which spelling errors I made and corrected while writing the text in front of you.

Handling inconsistent information

Data may have been entered correctly, but the respondent has filled in the questionnaire inconsistently. A respondent might claim to be male and pregnant or to be 23 with her oldest son being 19 years old.

Some researchers code all inconsistent data as missing, without further considerations. Others believe that the investigator should examine other information available and judge which piece of information is most likely to be correct. I recommend that you follow the latter principle — with caution. But no matter which principle you follow, you will have made a decision on how to interpret data, and such decisions must be documented in writing.

The missing-data problem

A nonresponse is a nonresponse, but in certain cases, missing data have a high cost. In a regression analysis with 10 predictors, an observation is omitted from the analysis if just one predictor is missing. If many observations have one or more missing predictors, this leads to a heavy loss of information — and the result may be biased if nonresponse is related to one of the factors of interest.

There are formal remedies for this situation. One remedy is missing-value imputation, where the most likely response is estimated from the characteristics of respondents with valid information; see [D] **impute**. There are some pitfalls to this solution, and the standard precondition of independence of observations is violated.

Sometimes you can make a reasonable judgment about missing data. For example, a woman whose children are 1, 9, and 20 years old is likely to be close to 40 herself. What is most correct: to consider her age unknown or to use 40 as a pretty close but imperfect judgment? If a respondent did not answer a question about a rare symptom, what is most correct: to treat it as no information or to consider it a "No"?

No matter what you decide, you must document your decision in writing.

Merging datasets

If you have several sources of data, make sure that all corrections have been made before merging; it is much more difficult to correct afterward.

```
───────────────── gen_visit12.do ─────────────────
* gen_visit12.do
* Merge corrected visit1c and visit2c datasets.
cd C:\docs\disx
use visit1c.dta
merge id using visit2c.dta, sort
save visit12.dta

tab1 _merge
list id _merge if _merge<3
```

Check that `merge` worked as intended (examine `_merge`; see section 9.5). Any unexpected mismatches might be due to errors in the matching variable (`id`) entered in one of the datasets, and such errors can be difficult to disentangle. Use the `duplicates report` command (see section 9.5) to check before merging whether the values of the matching variable are unique.

18.7   Modifying data

You should certainly not modify your original data, but you will often want to derive new variables from the original information. You might combine the information from several questions about well-being into one new variable or calculate the age from two dates and create 5-year age groups. When modifying data, follow these rules:

1. If you modify your data, save the result as a file with a new name that indicates the version (e.g., include a, b, or c, or 1, 2, or 3 in the filename).

2. Save the do-file containing the modifications with an appropriate name. I recommend using the gen prefix to illustrate that this do-file generates a new dataset.

3. Start the do-file with the command indicating the input data and end with the command indicating the output data. Omit commands that are not relevant to the modifications from the do-file.

4. Include comments to explain (to yourself or others) the purpose of complex operations.

5. Include further documentation (if needed) in the dataset by using the `label` and `note` commands.

`gen_visit12a.do` is the do-file generating `visit12a.dta`. It starts with the command reading the data (`use`) and ends with the command saving the modified data (`save`). The `cd` command is used to make sure that the datasets are located as intended.

```
┌──────────────────────── gen_visit12a.do ────────────────────────┐
* gen_visit12a.do
* generates visit12a.dta with new variables.

cd C:\docs\disx
use visit12.dta

* Calculate hrqol: quality of life score.
egen hrqol=rowsum(q1-q10)
label variable hrqol "Quality of life score"

* Calculate opage: age at operation.
generate opage=(opdate-bdate)/365.25
label variable opage "Age at operation"

* Calculate opagr: age groups at operation.
recode opage (55/max=4 "55+")(35/55=3 "35-54")(15/35=2 "15-34") ///
   (min/15=1 "-14"), generate(opagr)
label variable opagr "Age at operation, 4 groups"

label data "Visit12a.dta created by gen_visit12a.do, 02 jan 2004"
save visit12a.dta
```

Three new variables were created from the original information. To keep the original opage unchanged, I let the recode command generate the new variable opagr. You will want to define variables and value labels immediately after creating a new variable (you can do so within the recode command). It will never be easier than now, and it will make it much easier to read the do-file later.

Comments are helpful for explaining the purpose of complex operations.

label data attaches a label to the dataset to be displayed each time it is opened. Notes can be included in the dataset (note). You can display the notes included in a dataset by using the command notes; see section 7.1.

To make sure nothing unforeseen happens to your dataset, you can use the datasignature command; see [D] **datasignature**. Once you have arrived at what you believe is the final version of your dataset, include a datasignature set before the final save command as shown in the do-file above. This creates a signature, which is a function of the values of the variables and their names, and you can later check whether the data are consistent with the signature. The following illustrates the use of datasignature:

```
. sysuse auto.dta
(1978 Automobile Data)

. datasignature set
  74:12(71728):3831085005:1395876116        (data signature set)

. datasignature confirm
  (data unchanged since 10jun2007 14:31)
```

```
. replace price = . in 15
(1 real change made, 1 to missing)

. datasignature confirm
  data have changed since 10jun2007 14:31
r(9);

. datasignature set
  data signature already set -- specify option -reset-
r(110);

. datasignature set, reset
  74:12(71728):2350353367:3930547464        (data signature reset)
```

Check correctness of modifications

Errors do occur, and your modifications might not do what you intended. The modified do-file should demonstrate by your comments what you intended to do and by the commands what you actually did. Look at the distributions of the new variables, and list a sample of observations with both the source and target variables to check the correctness of calculations. By all means, print the lists before inspection! Reading on the screen is unreliable (and unpleasant, to say the least).

```
. use visit12a.dta

. codebook hrqol opage opagr, compact

. tab1 opagr

. sample 1

. slist q1-q10 hrqol

. sort opage

. list bdate opdate opage opagr
```

In the codebook output, look for the number of valid observations and for minimum and maximum values. tab1 is useful for variables with few categories, like opagr. The last commands are performed on a 1% sample only. slist lets you compare hrqol with the original values of q1-q10 and the derived age variables with the original dates. (slist works better than list with many variables. You can find and download it with findit slist; see section 10.2.) Sorting by opage makes the comparisons between opage and opagr easier.

If you identify inconsistencies, you must go back, modify gen_visit12a.do, and check again.

18.8 Analysis

Make sure you use the right dataset

For analyses beyond the simplest, I recommend using do-files, starting with the command that reads the data. There are two reasons for this recommendation:

1. You might, during a session, have made temporary modifications to your data (e.g., a selection of cases, or recoding a variable) and forgot that you did that.

2. Documenting an analysis includes documenting which dataset you used.

```
—————————————————— regress_sbp.do ——————————————————
* regress_sbp.do

cd C:\docs\disx
use visit12a.dta

regress sbp sex
regress sbp sex weight
regress sbp sex weight height
predict psbp
rvfplot, yline(0)
lincom _cons + 1*sex + 175*height + 80*weight
```

Late discovery of errors and inconsistencies

Despite your efforts to secure data quality, you may, during analysis, discover errors and inconsistencies. It is an obvious advantage to correct all errors before analysis, but if you organized your do-files, corrections are not that difficult. Go back and modify the correction do-file (gen_visit1c.do; section 18.6). Run this and the subsequent do-files, and you have a corrected analysis file. If you followed the recommendations in section 18.4 (log book, naming of do-files, a master do-file), this is easy. If not, the procedure will be time-consuming and prone to error.

18.9   Backing up and archiving

The distinction between backing up and archiving may seem subtle, but the purposes are different. *Backing up* is an everyday activity, and its purpose is to allow you to restore your data and documents in case of destruction or loss of data. Destruction may be physical, but most cases of data loss are due to human errors, such as unintentionally deleting or overwriting files.

Archiving takes place once or a few times during the life of a project. The purpose is to preserve your data and documents for a more distant future or maybe even to allow other researchers access to the information.

The computer professionals I know are trustworthy people, but their occupational mobility is high. Ask your supervisor or department if there is a local policy on issues of data protection, ownership of data, and responsibility for proper managing, backing up, and archiving data. Unfortunately, in many departments, these issues are not as clearly stated as they should be — in writing. If the department has no written instructions, take the full responsibility yourself. If there are instructions, evaluate them and decide if you need any further safeguards.

Backing up data

Strategy considerations

The way you handle your own data greatly affects your ability to back up and restore your data. I will especially point to the following issues:

- Use a logical and transparent folder structure, which is good for your everyday work — and makes it easier to back up and recover your data. Chapter 21 suggests a folder structure where your own data and documents are kept separately from program folders. All of your "own" files are located in subfolders under your main folder (C:\docs in this book).

- Back up not only datasets but also do-files modifying your data and written documents: protocol, codebook, log book, and other documenting information.

By far the safest strategy is to regularly back up all your files by using a semiautomated procedure.

Do a *full backup* with regular intervals, e.g., every 6 months. This backup includes all your data and documents — but not program files.

Take an *incremental backup* regularly, e.g., at the end of each working day. Include all new files and any files modified since the last backup.

Filenames are important. I recommend that you give your backup files names that enable you to sort them by age: 200512191723.zip for a zip file created at 5:23 P.M. on 19 December 2005. If you need to restore your data, start with the oldest to avoid overwriting new files with older versions.

Software considerations

There are several software options to consider. A good compression program is useful for backing up — and for other purposes, as well. I created the bkup command, which makes an incremental or full backup from a folder of your choice (e.g., C:\docs), including subfolders, to a compressed zip file with the name structure shown above. You can download bkup from this book's web site. It requires that the WinZip compression program be installed on your computer; you can read more in the accompanying help file (help bkup).

Media considerations

It is important that you store your backup media in a building other than the one where your computer resides; otherwise, in case of fire you may lose all data.

Diskettes are cheap but not very stable. If you rely on diskettes, you should make two copies to be stored separately.

CD-ROMs and *DVDs* are quite stable, provided you store them carefully, but the experience with long-term stability is limited.

Magnetic tape is probably history by now; stability varies.

Sending to a remote computer is my main recommendation; it requires no hardware beyond an Internet connection. If you have access to a server (located in a different building), you might use it for storing your backup files. If not, you may use, e.g., Google's Gmail facilities. Or you might have a mutual agreement with a friend living elsewhere to exchange backup files by email. Security and privacy considerations might lead you to encrypt the backup files; see later in this section.

Test your backup copy

Make sure that you actually can restore the data from your backup. If you use diskettes, CDs, or tapes, you must test them on a different computer, as the drives on other computers may differ in calibration.

Archiving

What to archive?

Whereas backing up is an everyday activity, archiving takes place once or a few times during the life of a project. If you used consistent documentation procedures with your data, then archiving is easy. If not, it is difficult. The final archiving of a project should include the following:

- Study protocol.

- Applications to and permissions from ethical review boards, etc.

- Data-collection instruments (e.g., questionnaires, case-report forms).

- Coding instructions and other technical descriptions.

- The log book (see section 18.4) and other written documentation on the processing of data.

- At least the first and the final version of your data.

- All do-files that modify data. The do-files should enable reconstruction of the final version from the first version of your data.

- Publications.

Where?

Archiving research data should be institutionalized, either by a research institution or a public or private agency. Opportunities vary, but there is an increasing understanding of the need for such an institution. The opportunities in Denmark are an excellent model.

The Danish State Archives has a division for storing electronic information, Danish Data Archive (http://www.dda.dk), which offers safe archiving of research data at no cost. The level of access is determined by the investigator, who can decide that she only has access herself, that others can get access with her permission, or that the data are accessible to anybody. The major Danish research funds request that data be archived at Danish Data Archive at the end of a project.

If you are affiliated with a research institution, it should take responsibility for the archiving of data—ask for written guidelines. However, many health researchers do not have a stable affiliation with a research institution, and that increases the need for some central organization.

Archiving data and keeping them readable is an active process where data are transformed to media and kept in current formats. In my department's basement, we, until recently, stored 8" and 5 1/4" floppy disks, magnetic tapes in various sizes, and even boxes with punch cards. To read them, we would probably need the help of a technical museum.

When?

There is no point in archiving undocumented data. Remember that archiving means storing for future use—in contrast to backup, which ensures viability of data in the short term. But waiting until completion and publication of the study can give you trouble; at that time, it can be difficult to collect the documents describing the process and to remember the computers on which the different versions of the data and do-files are kept.

The appropriate time for archiving depends on the project, but in general a two-step strategy is advisable:

1. Archive the raw dataset when you have finished entering data, corrected errors, and documented the data (see sections 18.6–18.7). Include all important documents, and archive copies of both data and the do-files that document modifications to data.
2. After analysis, archive updated data files and the corresponding do-files. Include copies of publications and other major documents written since the last archiving.

Isn't it difficult?

Archiving need not be difficult. If you have worked consistently with your data, you just need to archive the first and last datasets and the do-files documenting the modifications. If not, archiving is difficult—perhaps impossible.

18.10   Protecting against abuse

Motives and opportunities

Obviously sensitive information about people must be kept confidential without giving other people the opportunity to see the information.

The *motives* for intruding could be curiosity (my neighbor's mystery disease), economic gain (should we insure Mr. Smith?), creation of newspaper headlines ("Researchers fool around with confidential data"), and other indecent motives (if it becomes known that my colleague handles his data carelessly he will get in trouble—and I would love that).

It is the obligation of the researcher to give no other person the *opportunity* to see confidential information. Below I show two key methods to prevent unauthorized access to confidential electronic information.

Securing the electronic information is not enough. Information on paper must also be protected against unauthorized access. Information on paper is more vulnerable to accidental access than the information in a computer file.

Remove external identifiers

To link the source documents (e.g., questionnaires) with the dataset, you usually give each person a unique number also to be recorded in the dataset. This number is an internal identifier that has no meaning outside your project, as opposed to external identifiers (e.g., name, social security number). While analyzing, you usually do not need to keep any external identifiers in the dataset, so you should remove them.

Removing an external identifier is simple. For example:

```
───────────────────────── gen_safe_keyfile.do ─────────────────────────
* gen_safe_keyfile.do removes external identifier

cd C:\docs\disx
use unsafe.dta
keep intid extid
save a:\keyfile.dta

use unsafe.dta, clear
drop extid
save safe.dta


* When you have made sure that both files are valid:
erase unsafe.dta
```

The key file (`keyfile.dta`) linking the internal identifier (`intid`) with the external identifier (`extid`) should be encrypted and stored separately, i.e., not on the same computer as the information. It might be a good idea to store the key file at an archiving facility. Here I used a diskette, but know that diskettes are not very stable, so make an extra backup copy.

If you later need to include `extid`, such as for matching with external data, you can perform the following:

```
——————————————— gen_unsafe.do ———————————————
* gen_unsafe.do adds external identifier to data

cd C:\docs\disx
use safe.dta
sort intid
merge intid using a:\keyfile.dta, sort

save unsafe.dta
```

Encryption

There are several possibilities for encryption; I use the WinZip compression program and at the same time save disk space. It is easy and fast—but of course, you must neither forget your encryption password nor enable others to read it.

19 Appendix: Manuals and other good books

19.1 Stata manuals

The complete set of manuals comprises 17 volumes, but most users can make do with less. Although this list could be made in several ways, I list the manuals with those most relevant to health researchers first. You can see more information about the manuals at http://www.stata.com/bookstore/overview.html.

[GS]   *Getting Started.* Separate manuals based on the operating system: [GSW] for Windows, [GSM] for Macintosh, and [GSU] for Unix.

[I]   *Quick Reference and Index.* Will help you find your way through the documentation.

[U]   *User's Guide.* Gives a systematic overview and description of the Stata language, as well as many useful hints.

[D]   *Data Management Reference Manual.* Includes all commands relevant to calculation and other data-management commands. The content roughly matches chapters 8 and 9 of this book.

[R]   *Base Reference Manual.* Includes three volumes containing the bulk of Stata commands, except those in [D] and some other specialized commands that are described in the manuals listed below.

[G]   *Graphics Reference Manual.* Describes the commands to produce graphs.

[ST]   *Survival Analysis and Epidemiological Tables Reference Manual.* Devoted to survival analysis. Also, some other analyses frequently used in epidemiology (Mantel–Haenszel analysis) are included. The content roughly matches chapters 12 and 14 of this book.

[TS]   *Time-Series Reference Manual.* Includes commands and other tools for time-series analysis.

[XT]   *Longitudinal/Panel-Data Reference Manual.* Devoted to analysis of repeated measurements, as in panel studies.

[SVY]   *Survey Data Reference Manual.* Devoted to analysis of complex survey data. Includes discussions of poststratification, linearization, balanced repeated replication, and jackknife variance estimation methods.

[MV]   *Multivariate Statistics Reference Manual.* Includes several multivariate tech-
       niques, such as cluster analysis, factor analysis, principal component analysis,
       and correspondence analysis.

[P]   *Programming Reference Manual.* Includes several commands typically used
       in programs (ado-files).

[M]   *Mata Reference Manual.* Contains a systematic description of the matrix pro-
       gramming language, Mata, introduced with the version 9 release of Stata.

19.2   Other books about Stata

An increasing number of books about Stata and books using Stata to illustrate epidemiological
and biostatistical methods are being published. The best place to look for books about Stata is
Stata's own bookstore at http://www.stata.com/bookstore/. Take a look now, and then revisit for
new titles and new editions of existing books.

I have no intent to assess each of the books listed below, but I selected books of specific
interest primarily to health researchers.

Hamilton, L. C. 2006. *Statistics with Stata. Updated for version 9.* Belmont, CA: Brooks/Cole.

Rabe-Hesketh, S., and B. Everitt. 2007. *A Handbook of Statistical Analysis Using Stata.* 4th
     ed. Boca Raton, FL: Chapman & Hall/CRC.

Hills, M., and B. L. De Stavola. 2007. *A Short Introduction to Stata for Biostatistics.* London:
     Timberlake Consultants Press.

Cleves, M., W. Gould, R. G. Gutierrez, and Y. Marchenko. 2008. *An Introduction to Survival
     Analysis Using Stata.* 2nd ed. College Station, TX: Stata Press.

Long, J. S., and J. Freese. 2006. *Regression Models for Categorical Dependent Variables Using
     Stata.* 2nd ed. College Station, TX: Stata Press.

Mitchell, M. 2008. *A Visual Guide to Stata Graphics.* 2nd ed. College Station, TX: Stata Press.

19.3   Books using Stata

Several epidemiological and biostatistical textbooks use Stata more or less directly. Among my
favorites are the following:

Kirkwood, B. R., and J. A. C. Sterne. 2003. *Essential Medical Statistics.* 2nd ed. Malden, MA:
     Blackwell Science.

     The book is pretty close in its priorities to this book. Stata commands and output are not
     presented directly, but the Stata datasets used are available at
     http://www.blackwellpublishing.com/essentialmedstats/datasets.htm.

Dupont, W. D. 2002. *Statistical Modeling for Biomedical Researchers.* Cambridge: Cambridge University Press.

 The book includes many Stata examples, and the datasets used are available at http://www.mc.vanderbilt.edu/prevmed/wddtext/index.html#datasets.

Campbell, M. J. 2006. *Statistics at Square Two.* 2nd ed. Oxford: BMJ Books.

 The analyses in the book were performed using Stata, and typical Stata output is presented.

20 Appendix: Exercises

The following exercises are intended to help a beginner get started. Responses and comments to the exercises are not included in the book but in the file `exercise-comments.pdf`, which can be downloaded from the book's web site together with datasets and do-files. See the section about online supplements, page xviii. If you are a teacher using the book, you are welcome to use the exercises as course material.

Before starting, you must have prepared your Stata installation:

1. If you have not yet installed Stata, do it now (section 1.1).

2. If you have not yet updated Stata, do it now (section 1.1).

3. If you have not done so already, organize Stata's windows as shown in section 1.4. Once you have the windows organized as you desire, save your preferences by clicking on

   Edit ▷ Preferences ▷ Manage Preferences ▷ Save Preferences

4. Make a decision about which folder you want to use for the exercises related to this book. In the book's examples, it is `C:\docs\ishr2`, assuming that `C:\docs` is your personal main folder, but you may, of course, decide on another location. Find some more-detailed advice about folder structure in chapter 21.

   In Windows, use Explorer or My Computer to create the folder for exercises. You may also do it with Stata commands, as described in section 6.1:

   ```
   . cd C:\docs
   . mkdir ishr2
   . cd ishr2
   ```

5. At http://www.stata-press.com/data/ishr2.html, you will find instructions on how to download the datasets and do-files used in this book. To download the files to `C:\docs\ishr2`, type

   ```
   . cd C:\docs\ishr2
   . net from http://www.stata-press.com/data/ishr2/
   . net install ishr2-ado
   . net get ishr2-data
   . net get ishr2-do
   ```

   If you installed the files from the previous edition of this book, you will need to append the `replace` option to the `net install` command.

To see which files were downloaded, display the file list in the Results window by typing the Stata command

```
. dir
```

20.1   The user interface

The purpose of these first exercises is to help you get familiar with the user interface. You can find most of the information needed in sections 1.4 and 1.5.

20.1-1 In the Command window, type

```
. sysuse auto.dta
```

The `sysuse` command reads a dataset that is installed with Stata. Commands must be entered in lowercase; Stata does not understand `Sysuse` or `SYSUSE`. The initial period is Stata's command prompt. In Stata output, the prompt distinguishes commands from the rest of the output. You should not type the command prompt.

Look at the Variables window; it displays the names of variables in the `auto.dta` dataset.

20.1-2 Open the Data Browser by typing the command

```
. browse
```

and take a look. You might want to modify the window size or the font.

Now close the Data Browser. Open it again to see the values of `make`, `mpg`, and `foreign` for the first five observations by typing

```
. browse make mpg foreign in 1/5
```

`make` (a string variable) is displayed in red, while the value labels for `foreign` are displayed in blue. Right-click somewhere in the Data Browser window to toggle between value labels and codes for `foreign`.

You can also click on a button to open the Data Browser: . With the button, you will not be able to select which observations and variables to display, as you can with the `browse` command.

20.1-3 In the Command window, type

```
. summarize
```

and look at the Results window. `summarize` displays the number of valid observations, and the mean, standard deviation, and minimum and maximum values of all variables.

Use the mouse to highlight the table, and print it. (Click on the Print button or right-click and select Print.... In the dialog that appears, click on the Selection radio button.)

20.1-4 Look at the Review window, which displays the two commands issued so far (and possibly some errors you made). Now click on the last command (summarize) to copy it to the Command window (it must be a single click; a double-click executes the command instead). In the Variables window, click on mpg to copy it to the Command window, which now displays

> . summarize mpg

Press the *Enter* key and see what happens.

20.1-5 Try using the dialog system to obtain the same result. If you know the command name, you can access its dialog by typing

> . db *command_name*

For summarize, it would be

> . db summarize

If you are searching for a command but do not know its name, use the menu system. For summarize, select

> Statistics ▷ Summaries, tables, and tests ▷
> Summary and descriptive statistics ▷ Summary statistics

In the dialog that appears, use the drop-down list in the Variables field and select mpg. Click on the OK button.

The dialogs generate commands. For summarize mpg, it obviously is easier to type the command than to create it by using the dialog, but for complex commands and graphs, the dialogs are an advantage. In this book, I rarely describe how to use a dialog. Instead, I show commands which you can enter by using the Command window, a do-file, or the dialog system.

20.1-6 Click anywhere in the Review window, and press *Ctrl+A* to select all commands. Then press *Ctrl+C* to copy them to the Windows Clipboard. Now open the Do-file Editor; you can do it by clicking on the Do-file Editor button, , or by typing the command

> . doedit

Next paste the selected commands to the Do-file Editor by pressing *Ctrl+V*. Edit the text so that the Do-file Editor now contains only these three lines:

> . sysuse auto.dta
> . summarize
> . summarize mpg

Save the revised do-file as test1.do. Make sure it is saved in C:\docs\ishr2 (or wherever you prefer). Now click on the Do-file Editor's Do button, , and see what happens. In the Results window, you will see output like the following:

```
. do "C:\Temp\STD00000000.tmp"

. sysuse auto.dta
(1978 Automobile Data)

. summarize
    Variable |      Obs       Mean   Std. Dev.      Min        Max
-------------+--------------------------------------------------------
        make |        0
       price |       74   6165.257   2949.496       3291      15906
         mpg |       74    21.2973   5.785503         12         41
```
(output omitted)

Instead of the output above, you might see something like this:

```
. sysuse auto.dta
no; data in memory would be lost
r(4);
```

This happens if the data in memory have been modified but not saved. It is a safeguard against loss of data. If you are certain that the data in memory need not be saved, you can type the command

```
. clear
```

in the Command window and, in the Do-file Editor, click on the Do button again.

This process was easy, but the name of the do-file was not displayed. To document your work better, try instead to execute it from the Command window:

```
. do "C:\docs\ishr2\test1.do"
```

Instead of specifying the full path for each file, you can specify the file path by using the cd command (see section 6.1):

```
. cd "c:\docs\ishr2"
. do "test1.do"
```

Rather than remembering the exact path and name of the do-file, it may be easier to find it by selecting

File ▷ Do...

20.2   Managing output

The following exercises relate to sections 1.6 and 1.7 and are designed to give you some experience with methods of handling the output.

20.2-1 Make clear to yourself in which folder you are working (look in the lower-left corner of the main Stata window). If you need to change folders, do that.

Open an output log (text format):

```
. log using stata.log
```

If there is already a `stata.log` file in the current folder, your request will be rejected:

```
. log using stata.log
file c:\docs\ishr2\stata.log already exists
r(602);
```

Dependent upon what you want, you must either type

```
. log using stata.log, append
```

or

```
. log using stata.log, replace
```

For now, I suggest the `replace` option; then you start on a new output log.

20.2-2 Do a few things with the `auto.dta` dataset (see the exercises in section 20.1) to create some output to work with. Next click on the Log button, 🗔 , or press *Ctrl+L* and select View snapshot of log file. The output (`stata.log`) from the entire session is now displayed in a Viewer window. Here you can use the mouse to select what you want to print, but you cannot edit anything. Also try to copy parts of the output to your word processor. Use a fixed-width font, e.g., Courier, to make tables align correctly.

20.2-3 Close the log and open a new log, now with the SMCL format:

```
. log close
. log using stata.smcl
```

Again, do a few things with the `auto.dta` dataset to create some output. One suggestion would be

```
. describe
. regress mpg weight
```

Display this log in the Viewer. What differences do you note?

20.2-4 You may want, like me, to let Stata open an output log file automatically at session start, to collect all output. A `profile.do` is mentioned in section 1.6, and a more elaborate version is shown in section 17.5. If you downloaded the files belonging to the book, the elaborate `profile.do` was included. Copy it to `C:\ado\personal` (create the folder if it does not exist already).

The commands in `profile.do` will be executed next time you start Stata.

20.3 Calculations

The purpose of this exercise is to gain experience with various calculation procedures. Most of the commands are explained in chapter 8; the documentation commands (`label`, etc.), in chapter 7; and the `use` and `save` commands, in chapter 6.

We use the `smoke.dta` dataset; it is one of the datasets available at this book's web site; see item 5 in the introduction to chapter 20. The dataset includes these variables:

Variable	Meaning	Possible values
id	ID number	1–250
sex	Sex	1 male
		2 female
age	Age (years)	0–99
weight	Weight (kg)	40–150
height	Height (cm)	100–250
smoker	Smoker?	0 no
		1 current smoker
		2 former smoker
cigaret	Cigarettes per day	0–99
cheroot	Cigars or cheroots per day	0–99
pipe	Packs of pipe tobacco per week	0–9

20.3-1 In the Command window, enter (provided you copied the files to C:\docs\ishr2)

```
. cd "C:\docs\ishr2"
. use smoke.dta
. codebook, compact
```

Inspect the codebook output. What does it mean that there are fewer observations for weight and height than for the other variables?

Do the minimum and maximum values give rise to any suspicion of errors?

Instead of codebook, compact, you could use summarize; try that. What is the difference in output from these two commands? (With large datasets, summarize is faster than codebook, compact.)

20.3-2 Say you are going to publish your results in an American journal that wants the results presented as inches and pounds (lb.) rather than centimeters (cm) and kilograms (kg). One inch is 2.54 cm, and one lb. is 0.454 kg. Create the new variables weightlb (weight in lb.) and heightin (height in inches).

Study the output from a new codebook, compact command, and consider whether the results look right. Also make relevant calculations (by paper and pencil or by a hand-held calculator) to check the results.

Instead of a hand-held calculator, try using the display command (see section 10.6).

20.3-3 The two new variables should be furnished with variable labels; do that (see chapter 7). Give a new codebook, compact command to see if it worked as intended.

20.3-4 The body mass index (BMI) is defined as weight (kg) divided by height squared (height in meters). Generate the new variable bmi, furnish it with a label, and check the result.

20.3-5 Save the revised dataset, including the three new variables weightlb, heightin, and bmi, to the hard disk as smoke1.dta (see section 6.1). Because this leads to a new version of the dataset, it is strongly recommended to do it in a do-file, starting with

```
. cd "C:\docs\ishr2"      (or wherever your data are stored)
. use smoke.dta
```

and ending with

```
. save smoke1.dta
```

with the calculation and labeling commands between the use and save commands. Find examples of such do-files in sections 7.2 and 18.7.

You may get this error message:

```
. use smoke.dta
no; data in memory would be lost
r(4);
```

What does it mean, and what can you do about it?

You may get this error message:

```
. save smoke1.dta
file smoke1.dta already exists
r(602);
```

What does it mean, and what can you do about it?

Did you save the do-file creating smoke1.dta? What name did you give it? (My recommendation is gen_smoke1.do, the do-file that generates smoke1.dta; see section 18.4).

20.3-6 Create a new variable, agegrp, which is a reasonable grouping of age (see recode, section 8.4). Before deciding the groups, look at the summarize or codebook output, and look at the minimum and maximum values. Define the variable label and value labels for the new variable (label variable, label define, label values; see chapter 7). The smartest thing to do is to include the commands in the do-file from question 20.3-5, before the save command, and run the do-file again. Check that the result is as intended; see an example in section 8.4.

20.3-7 Create a new variable, tobacco, which is tobacco use in grams per day (1 cigarette = 1 g, 1 cigar/cheroot = 2 g, 1 pack of pipe tobacco = 40 g). (Use generate; see section 8.1.) Define an informative variable label for tobacco (label variable; see chapter 7). Again, include the commands needed in gen_smoke1.do.

20.3-8 From smoke1.dta, see a frequency table for tobacco (tab1; see section 10.3). Compare with the frequency tables for cigaret, etc., and decide if the result makes sense. Also list the first 30 observations to see if you obtained the result intended (on listing, see section 10.2):

```
. list cigaret cheroot pipe tobacco in 1/30
```

If there are errors, make corrections in gen_smoke1.do and run it again.

20.3-9 This exercise is about precision problems. I suggest reading section 5.4. Give these commands and study the output carefully:

```
. clear
. set obs 1
. generate x1 = 1/5
. generate double x2 = 1/5
. list
. list if x1 == 0.2
. list if x2 == 0.2
```

The second `list` command produced no output. What happened?

20.4   Working with missing values

I suggest reading section 5.3 on missing values.

20.4-1 Use the `smoke1x.dta` dataset downloaded from the book's web site or the `smoke1.dta` dataset generated in exercise 20.3-5. Make a list of all whose BMI is larger than 30, showing the variables `id`, `weight`, `height`, and `bmi` (`list` with the `if` qualifier). Study the list carefully; there may be surprises.

20.4-2 Enter the following commands in the Do-file Editor, execute the commands, and study the list output.

```
set obs 1
generate a = 1/0
generate b = sqrt(-4)
generate c = ln(0)
generate d = mdy(2,29,2001)
generate e = a+5
list
```

If the result is a missing value, what is the reason in each case?

20.5   Working with date variables

I suggest reading section 5.5 on date and time variables. In these exercises, we will work with date variables only, not with time variables.

20.5-1 Use the `dates.dta` dataset, which can be downloaded from the book's web site. It is a small dataset with three observations. The information on the date of birth is stored in three numeric variables, and the information on an admission date is stored in a string variable with the sequence day, month, year:

```
. cd C:\docs\ishr2

. use dates.dta

. describe

Contains data from dates.dta
  obs:              3
  vars:             4                          18 Jan 2008 17:08
  size:            78 (99.9% of memory free)

              storage  display   value
variable name   type   format    label    variable label

bd            float    %9.0g              Day of birth
bm            float    %9.0g              Month of birth
by            float    %9.0g              Year of birth
adate_s       str10    %10s               Date of admission (string)

Sorted by:
```

Generate a new version, dates2.dta, including two date variables, one for the date of birth and one for the date of admission, and a variable with the age of admission for each person. Obviously, this should be done with a do-file. list the result and examine it.

20.5-2 Modify the display format for the birth date variable so that 12 March 1955 is displayed as 03/12/1955.

20.5-3 What is the numeric value of the date 1 July 2008? (Hint: Use display [see section 10.6] in combination with the mdy() function.)

What date has the numeric value 2345? (Hint: Use display with the %td format specification.)

20.6   Description and simple analysis

For the following questions, use the smoke1.dta dataset created in the preceding section, or—if you did not do that—use smoke1x.dta, which can be downloaded from the book's web site. You can find most of the relevant commands in chapter 10.

20.6-1 Make overviews of the dataset with the describe, codebook, and summarize commands. Compare the outputs, and make clear to yourself the similarities and differences.

20.6-2 Make a simple table of smoker (tab1). If you miss the numerical codes, try

```
. numlabel, add
```

and run the tab1 command again. What happened? (On numlabel, see section 7.1.) Actually, you want the display of both code and value label to be in effect in future analyses from this dataset. Include the numlabel command in gen_smoke1.do, and run it again.

20.6-3 Describe with a cross-tabulation the joint age and sex distribution of the study population (tab2; see section 10.3). Would you prefer the original age or the grouped age for this kind of table? Include percentages in the table to show the relative age distribution for each sex, and perform a chi-squared test and Fisher's exact test.

20.6-4 Make two tables describing the average BMI by sex and by age groups (oneway or tabstat or table; see section 10.4). Test if the mean BMI is different for men and women (ttest; see section 10.4).

20.6-5 The *t* test in question 20.6-4 requires that the distribution of the dependent variable (bmi) is normal for each sex. Examine if this requirement is met for women (histogram, qnorm, swilk). Would a log transformation be relevant? If yes, try it (the ln() function; see section 8.2).

20.6-6 The *t* test in question 20.6-4 requires that the standard deviation of the dependent variable is not different for the compared groups. Examine if this requirement is fulfilled (sdtest).

20.6-7 Estimate the mean BMI with a 95% confidence interval. Estimate the proportion of males with a 90% confidence interval.

20.6-8 Section 10.6 shows the use of immediate commands. Try the examples or invent some similar examples.

20.7   Taking good care of your data

These exercises are do-file examples of how *not* to take good care of your data. Each do-file violates at least one of the recommendations about safe data handling in this book. Find and describe the problems, and suggest improvements. I suggest reading chapter 18.

20.7-1

```
───────────────── gen_xyz1.do ─────────────────
* gen_xyz1.do

cd "C:\docs\project xyz"
generate age1 = (date1 - bdate)/365.25
generate bmi = weight/(height^2)

* This do-file generated two new variables.
```

20.7-2

```
───────────────── gen_xyz1.do ─────────────────
* gen_xyz1.do

cd "C:\docs\project xyz"
use xyz1.dta
generate age1 = (date1 - bdate)/365.25
generate bmi = weight/(height^2)
keep if bmi < .
save xyz1.dta, replace
```

20.7-3

```
_____ gen_xyz1.do _____
* gen_xyz1.do

cd "C:\docs\project xyz"
use xyz1.dta
generate age1 = (date1 - bdate)/365.25
generate bmi = weight/(height^2)
save xyz2.dta
```

20.7-4

```
_____ gen_xyz1.do _____
* gen_xyz1.do

cd "C:\docs\project xyz"
use xyz.dta
generate age1 = (date1 - bdate)/365.25
recode age1 (min/20=1)(20/40=2)(40/max=3)
generate bmi = weight/(height^2)
save xyz1.dta
```

20.7-5

```
_____ gen_xyz2.do _____
* gen_xyz2.do

cd "C:\docs\project xyz"
use xyz1.dta
replace age1 = age1 - 5 if sex==2
replace bmi = bmi - 2 if sex==2
save xyz2.dta
```

20.7-6

```
_____ gen_xyz1.do _____
* gen_xyz1.do

cd "C:\docs\project xyz"
use xyz.dta

generate age1 = (date1 - bdate)/365.25
label variable age1 "Age at admission"

recode age1 (40/max=3)(20/40=2)(min/20=1), generate(age1grp)
label variable age1grp "Age (grouped) at admission"

generate bmi = weight/(height^2)
label variable bmi "Body mass index (kg/m^2)"

save xyz1.dta
```

20.7-7

```
──────────────────────── gen_xyz1.do ────────────────────────
* gen_xyz2.do

cd "C:\docs\project xyz"

use xyz.dta

generate age1 = (date1 - bdate)/365.25
label variable age1 "Age at admission"

recode age1 (40/max=3 "40+")(20/40=2 "20-39") (min/20=1 "-19") ,  ///
   generate(age1grp)
label variable age1grp "Age (grouped) at admission"

generate bmi = weight/(height^2)
label variable bmi "Body mass index (kg/m^2)"

save xyz1.dta
```

21 Appendix: Advice about working with Windows

This appendix includes some tools and advice about working with Windows. My main comments and recommendations apply to handling the folder (directory) structure. There are several ways to move and copy files; I show only one technique.

The techniques shown are a minimum of what you must be able to perform. Without them, you are at risk of creating accidents, either by losing important data or by being unable to locate them.

Create a smart folder structure

Do not mix your own data and documents with program files. To do so is risky and will inevitably lead to confusion. Create a personal main folder (the Documents folder), e.g., C:\docs, with all of your own files (data, do-files, text documents) in subfolders under the main folder. This approach will also facilitate backing up your data (see section 18.9). If you work in a networked setting, talk with your network administrator before restructuring things.

Your Windows installation may have placed your Documents folder somewhere along a long path under C:\Documents and Settings. This placement may complicate things for you, and I suggest (and, in this book, I assume in the examples) a simpler structure in which you make C:\docs your Documents folder.

First create the C:\docs folder (see *How to create a new folder* later in this appendix).

Next make C:\docs your default main folder. Click on [Start]. The appearance now depends on the Windows version you are using, but there should be an icon with the name Documents. Right-click on it and select **Properties**. Replace the current location of the default destination folder with C:\docs. When asked if you want to move folders and files from the current to the new location, click on **Yes**.

Organize your folder structure by subject, not by file type. Here is an example:

```
C:\
    ado
        personal
        plus
    docs
        ishr2
        Personal
            CV
            Secrets (encrypted)
        Project 1
            Protocol
            Administration
            Data
                Safe
            Manuscripts
        Project 2
            Protocol
            Administration
            Data
                Safe
            Manuscripts
    Program files
        EpiData
        Games
            Solitaire
            GTA
        OpenOffice
        Stata10
            ado
                base
                updates
        WinZip
    Windows
```

This structure has several advantages, such as the following:

- You avoid mixing your "own" files with program files.
- Your Documents folder (C:\docs) is the default root folder for all your own subfolders (the white area), and when opening and saving files, you will look primarily at these folders, not the program folders.
- It is much easier to set up a consistent backup procedure (see section 18.9).

If your hard disk is partitioned into a C: and a D: drive, using C:\ for programs and D:\ as your Documents folder is a good idea:

```
C:\
    ado
        personal
        plus
    Program files
        . . .
        Stata10
            ado
                base
                updates
        WinZip
    Windows
```

```
D:\
        ishr2
        Personal
            CV
            Secrets (encrypted)
    Project 1
        Protocol
        Administration
        Data
            Safe
        Manuscripts
    Project2
    . . .
```

How to select a default working folder for a program

The installation default working folder for many programs is the program folder itself. This default is an extremely poor choice, and you should never mix your own documents and data files with program files. You might never find your own files again, you might accidentally delete your data (such as when installing a new version of the program), or you might accidentally delete program files.

Stata initially suggests C:\data as the default working folder, which is a lot better, and it is okay when you are working with sample data. But as soon as you start working with real data, you should organize things by subject, not by programs. To define C:\docs as the default working folder for Stata, right-click on the Stata desktop icon, and select

Properties ▷ Shortcut ▷ Start in

and then type C:\docs.

Using Windows Explorer

I prefer using Explorer rather than My Computer. To put a shortcut on the desktop, find `explorer.exe` (typically in the `C:\Windows` folder). Right-click on `explorer.exe` and select

> Create shortcut

Make Windows display filename extensions

For reasons not understood by me, Microsoft decided not to display filename extensions by default. This choice is inconvenient (you cannot distinguish the do-file `alpha.do` from the dataset `alpha.dta`), so you should set Windows to display filename extensions. Open Windows Explorer and select

> Tools ▷ Folder options ▷ View

You will see several check boxes. Uncheck Hide extensions for known file types.

Creating a new folder

Let's create a new folder called `project3` under `C:\docs`:

- Double-click on the Explorer icon on the desktop.

- Click on `C:\docs` (root folder for own files).

- Select File ▷ New ▷ Folder.

- Rename "`New Folder`" to "`project3`".

You can also use Stata's `mkdir` command (see section 6.1) to create a new folder:

```
. cd c:\docs
. mkdir "project3"
```

Renaming a folder or file

- In Explorer, right-click on the folder or file, and select Rename.

- Type the name desired and press *Enter*.

Copying a file or a folder to another folder or to a diskette

- In Explorer, highlight the source file or folder, and press *Ctrl+C* (copy to clipboard).

- Highlight the target folder (or `A:`), and press *Ctrl+V* (paste from clipboard).

Stata's `copy` command performs the same functions (with some restrictions); see [D] **copy**.

How to move a file or a folder to another folder

- In Explorer, highlight the source file or folder icon, and press *Ctrl+X* (copy to clipboard and delete source file).

- Highlight the target folder and press *Ctrl+V* (paste from clipboard).

You can also copy or move files and folders by using the mouse to drag and drop. But be aware that the effect is different whether you drag and drop within the same medium (disk) or between media. The *Ctrl+C*, *Ctrl+X*, *Ctrl+V* method works consistently, and it works much the same as when you are editing text in a word processor or in Stata's Do-file Editor.

Write-protect your files

To prevent a file from accidental deletion or overwriting, you can write-protect it. To see the write-protection attribute for a file, right-click on the file in Explorer, and select **Properties**. You can change the write-protection manually.

Smart users write-protect their vital data and do-files once they are satisfied with them.

References

Altman, D. G. 1990. *Practical Statistics for Medical Research.* London: Chapman & Hall.

Bland, J. M. 2000. *An Introduction to Medical Statistics.* 3rd ed. Oxford: Oxford University Press.

Bland, J. M., and D. G. Altman. 1986. Statistical methods for assessing agreement between two methods of clinical measurement. *Lancet* I: 307–310.

———. 2003. Applying the right statistics: Analyses of measurement studies. *Ultrasound in Obstetrics and Gynecology* 22: 85–93.

Breslow, N. E., and N. E. Day. 1993. *Statistical Methods in Cancer Research: Volume 1 — The Analysis of Case–Control Studies.* Lyon, UK: International Agency for Research on Cancer.

Campbell, M. J. 2006. *Statistics at Square Two.* 2nd ed. Oxford: BMJ Books.

Clayton, D., and M. Hills. 1993. *Statistical Models in Epidemiology.* Oxford: Oxford University Press.

Cleves, M., W. Gould, R. G. Gutierrez, and Y. Marchenko. 2008. *An Introduction to Survival Analysis Using Stata.* 2nd ed. College Station, TX: Stata Press.

Coviello, V., and M. Boggess. 2004. Cumulative incidence estimation in the presence of competing risks. *Stata Journal* 4: 103–112.

Cox, N. J. 2003a. Speaking Stata: Problems with lists. *Stata Journal* 3: 185–202.

———. 2003b. Speaking Stata: Problems with tables, Part II. *Stata Journal* 3: 420–439.

———. 2004. Speaking Stata: Graphing model diagnostics. *Stata Journal* 4: 449–475.

———. 2005. Some notes on text editors for Stata users. http://fmwww.bc.edu/repec/bocode/t/textEditors.html.

Doll, R., and A. B. Hill. 1950. Smoking and carcinoma of the lung. Preliminary report. *BMJ* 2: 84–93.

Dupont, W. D. 2002. *Statistical Modeling for Biomedical Researchers: A Simple Introduction to the Analysis of Complex Data.* Cambridge: Cambridge University Press.

Egger, M., G. Davey Smith, and D. G. Altman. 2001. *Systematic Reviews in Health Care: Meta-Analysis in Context.* 2nd ed. London: BMJ Books.

Farley, T. M. M., M. M. Ali, and E. Slaymaker. 2001. Competing approaches to analysis of failure times with competing risks. *Statistics in Medicine* 20: 3601–3610.

Feiveson, A. H. 2001. FAQ: How can I use Stata to calculate power by simulation? http://www.stata.com/support/faqs/stat/power.html.

———. 2002. Power by simulation. *Stata Journal* 2: 107–124.

Habbema, J. D., R. Eijkemans, P. Krijnen, and J. A. Knottnerus. 2002. Analysis of data on the accuracy of diagnostic tests. In *The Evidence Base of Clinical Diagnosis*, 117–144. London: BMJ Books.

Hosmer, D. W., Jr., and S. Lemeshow. 2000. *Applied Logistic Regression*. 2nd ed. New York: Wiley.

Hosmer, D. W., Jr., S. Lemeshow, and S. May. 2008. *Applied Survival Analysis: Regression Modeling of Time to Event Data*. 2nd ed. New York: Wiley.

Juul, S. 2003. Lean mainstream schemes for Stata 8 graphics. *Stata Journal* 3: 295–301.

———. 2005. *Take Good Care of Your Data*. Aarhus: Institute of Public Health, University of Aarhus. http://www.folkesundhed.au.dk/uddannelse/software/takecare.pdf.

Kirkwood, B. R., and J. A. C. Sterne. 2003. *Essential Medical Statistics*. 2nd ed. Oxford: Blackwell Science.

Lindholt, J. S., S. Juul, H. Fasting, and E. W. Henneberg. 2005. Screening for abdominal aortic aneurysms: Single centre randomised controlled trial. *BMJ* 330: 750–752.

Metha, C. R., and N. R. Patel. 1995. Exact logistic regression: Theory and examples. *Statistics in Medicine* 14: 2143–2160.

Mitchell, M. 2008. *A Visual Guide to Stata Graphics*. 2nd ed. College Station, TX: Stata Press.

Newson, R. 2004. Generalized power calculations for generalized linear models and more. *Stata Journal* 4: 379–401.

Pepe, M. S. 2003. *The Statistical Evaluation of Medical Tests for Classification and Prediction*. Oxford: Oxford University Press.

Pocock, S. J., T. C. Clayton, and D. G. Altman. 2002. Survival plots of time-to-event outcomes in clinical trials: Good practice and pitfalls. *Lancet* 359: 1686–1689.

Robbins, N. B. 2005. *Creating More Effective Graphs*. Hoboken, NJ: Wiley.

Sackett, D. L., and R. B. Haynes. 2002. The architecture of diagnostic research. In *The Evidence Base of Clinical Diagnosis*, ed. J. A. Knottnerus. London: BMJ Books.

Sackett, D. L., R. B. Haynes, G. H. Guyatt, and P. Tugwell. 1991. *Clinical Epidemiology: A Basic Science for Clinical Medicine*. 2nd ed. Boston: Little, Brown and Company.

Tukey, J. W. 1977. *Exploratory Data Analysis*. Reading, MA: Addison–Wesley.

University Group Diabetes Program. 1970. A study of the effects of hypoglycemic agents on vascular complications in patients with adult onset diabetes. *Diabetes* 19: 747–830.

Author index

Subject index